The
H₂O DIET

How to Eat, Exercise, Drink and Dream

By

Gene Coates, M.A.
Jeannette Murueta, DDS

VISUAL CREDITS

Cover, "A Splash of Lime," .supernova.
Page 1, "Paradise," janusz 1
Page 11, "Fruits," GenkiGenki
Page 29, "Morning Falls on Chewacla," Laura Travels
Page 39, "Kumagaya fireworks festival #4," syuu
Page 49, "Cold Reception," jaxxon
Page 55, "Vancouver Bridge at Sunset," Stuck in Customs
Page 65, "Clouds over Deer Lake," Slack12
Page 75, "Merry-go-round," chatirygirl
Page 87, "NASA's Earth Observatory: the Blue Marble,"
        GISuser
Page 95, "What's your favorite?" Gúnna
Page 107, "Rainbow on the Water," guorui
Page 123, "Colors," canadianguy
Page 139, "Drops of roses," Steve took it
Page 155, "Shangri-la Mactan," bingbing
Page 165, "coffee," cygnoir
Page 179, "Breakfast fruit bowl," markus941
Page 182, "Glucose," Helen Coates
Page 182, "Sucrose," Helen Coates
Page 187, "Venècia-Venice," Mor (benbits)
Page 191, "Looks like the kids are bored again," whiskymac

Technical Consultants: John E. Coates, Helen J. Coates

Visit www.amazon.com to order additional copies

To our parents Eduardo, Bertha, Harry and Helen,
and our children Helen and John,
who inspired us to discover a new way.

iv

PREFACE

Many of us are desperate to redefine our lives, to get out of the rut of unhealthy eating and living, and make a new beginning. But we really do not have any idea where to begin. Unfortunately, amongst that sea of information and propaganda floating around out there, it daily becomes more difficult to separate the wheat from the chaff. This book is a determined effort to reduce the task of regaining control of our lives to the basics. We also were a bit too overweight, too fatigued both during and at the end of long days, and too stressed out to reorient ourselves. Let us share with you what we discovered.

Starting a new diet with no idea of the reasons behind the diet is a recipe for failure. In this book, we provide you with essential information about losing weight based on the nutritional needs of people in general, a realistic everyday exercise program, and a strategy to get rid of the extra weight permanently. This knowledge can be applied to anyone's diet without changing your essential personal preferences. Just the opposite: this information could allow you to eat the foods you like the most without having the secondary effect of gaining weight. The key element for your discovering the ideal structure for your diet is knowledge. Would making changes in your current diet make sense? Try and see for yourself.

"Our life is frittered away by detail…Simplify, simplify."

—Thoreau

Table of Contents

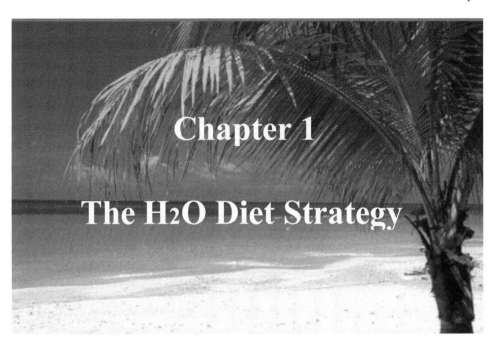

Chapter 1

The H₂O Diet Strategy

AN INFORMED WAY TO LOSE WEIGHT

A new season is coming in your life. Get ready to lose weight with the H₂O Diet. Do not let this opportunity to genuinely lose weight slip by. Little by little, you will see your weight disappear—in a permanent way. Give your body a break. Stop carrying around all those gallons of extra water. Yes, you heard correctly. The body retains the amount of water necessary to burn its accumulated fat. Just imagine yourself carting around an extra 2 or 3 gallons of water everywhere you go, a gallon jug dangling from each arm. Well, you probably are.

The H₂O Diet gives the opportunity to your body to burn the fat that has been accumulating for years. It is a sure and permanent way to lose weight. With our H₂O Diet, you gain control of your weight. You can work in close contact with the needs of your body, providing it with what it really needs. It is an informed way to lose the accumulated fat, and never let it accumulate in your body again.

Water is the main focus of this diet. If you do not drink enough water, your body will not have the water necessary to accomplish its basic functions. We need water for everything. But beware: moderation is key to all we do. Excessive consumption of water could prove to be fatal.

The main objective of the H2O Diet is to provide the amount of water that a person needs—on an individual basis— to maintain a perfect equilibrium in the body, which results in improved health. We have reviewed several diet books, observing that everyone seems to be overlooking one of the most important nutrients in everyone's diet: "water." Even the U.S. government's food pyramid does not have any information about the amount of water we require every day.

It seems that we take for granted that everyone knows how much water we should consume. Or maybe we are simply leaving the responsibility to our instincts. But let's not forget that we are being constantly brainwashed by advertising promoting so many competing products that we supposedly should be drinking, that we are virtually learning to ignore water. And it seems that no one is giving us information about what happens in our bodies every time we take a sip of soda or juice.

The H2O Diet gives you an essential orientation of how your body functions in utilizing carbohydrates and fats as sources of energy. Also, we will attempt to give you the information you need to get rid of that surplus fat you have accumulated in your body throughout the years. This is not a fast way to lose weight. Rather, this is a diet focused on discovering a natural equilibrium in your body to maintain health. And this equilibrium will allow your body to do the job it is optimally programmed to do, yet one that has been postponed for a long time. In fact, this will take some time. We won't provide you with a special diet. You will eat your normal diet, but will begin to substitute some starchy foods with enhanced portions of fruits and vegetables, which are obviously healthy, and necessary in order for your body to maintain its equilibrium while you are losing weight.

Many times the answer is right in front of us, yet we are unable to see it. For whatever reason, we are unable to focus in on certain things, unless we pay special attention. That is why companies advertise—to capture our attention, to make us focus on their products. But there are other things that, for some peculiar reason, get our attention. At times we are traumatized in the process. And this trauma makes us pay special attention to a subject. Once we pay attention, many times we discover that what seemed impossible to comprehend at the beginning, becomes easier to resolve later as we become familiar with the circumstances surrounding the subject. At times, the simplest element can be the solution to a complex problem. Let's not wait to be traumatized to get focused on this subject. Let's do something now!

As a nation, we are having this incredible problem with obesity and the illnesses that come with it. And that is traumatizing. Despite all the advertising about diets and ways to lose weight, it seems impossible for people to actually do it. We still see overweight people everywhere—even in our own mirrors. And here it is again: you won't lose weight being blind to the facts, and following someone else's diet. You have to focus your attention on the way your body functions, and investigate this process as thoroughly as you can. Each of us is unique in the way we eat, but similar to each other in the way our bodies function. Until you can really see the facts, and focus in on the information about the way your body works, and what it really needs, you are going to have a hard time losing weight. With modern agriculture and commerce, everything has changed. We have at our fingertips all kinds of foods in all seasons. But we have to become educated about the way we utilize them. Once you immerse yourself in this issue and become familiarized with it, it will seem incredible that you never had a 3-dimensional sense of it before.

The other day, we saw a report on TV that really impressed us. The mother of a six-year old boy that had just been diagnosed with diabetes was saying, "I would have done anything, anything, to prevent this from happening." This made us think more about the subject, and focus our attention more sharply, asking ourselves: what could have been done? We had been already thinking about the subject because we work in health care, and have witnessed young people being diagnosed with diabetes—people with no insurance, facing a lifetime illness. We made a decision. We would study the subject to find out if there was something that could be done.

We started to study the subject as thoroughly as we could. And now, we have concluded that the H2O Diet can help us to stay healthy. The information we need already exists. We just need to review it, and make decisions that will change our lives forever. We do not have to be overweight or obese. And possibly, if we are not overweight, like nutrition experts and doctors are saying, we will reduce the possibility of getting diabetes or other illnesses related to obesity. The H2O Diet is based on advice that our doctors recommend, but that we forget as soon as we leave the doctor's office. Our problem is that we do not focus enough. We do not know which facts to focus on in order to follow the medical advice. As people say, words go in one ear and out the other. At times, we follow the advice of the doctor for a few days while we are sick, and then forget completely, because we think that we only need to consciously drink water while we are sick. This brings into play another factor. Doctors often advise us to drink plenty of water when we are sick, but how much is plenty? Doctors need to educate their patients in this subject, and not assume that the word "plenty" delivers a satisfactory concept to the patient about how much water they should be drinking.

Now that we know that the H2O Diet is the answer to our questions, we feel that we have a serious responsibility. We need to tell other people about it. It took us decades to find out for ourselves, to focus properly on the subject. And we are aware that other people are in desperate need of this diet. We see them everywhere and we want to tell them. That is the reason why we decided to write this book. Our children also have benefited from knowing and utilizing this information, and support the idea of sharing this information. We want to see America changing direction. Now.

The core intent of the H2O Diet is to help people to stay healthy. Please, stay focused on this subject until you become familiar with it, as if your life depended on it.

THE BASICS

This book talks about the causes of obesity—the misunderstandings that make us store excessive fat, how to stop adding pounds, and start losing them.

The body normally stores the macronutrients fat, carbohydrates and protein, together with the water it needs to release their energy in case of normal demand, or emergency. That is why people can live several days without any food or water. It is for this reason that we can gain or lose so much weight in little time. When you burn carbohydrates, fat, or protein, the body releases water. The body does not like to accumulate too much of any of the sources of energy, because they can cause damage to the overall well being of the individual. It is for this reason that the body has several defense mechanisms to prevent that accumulation. For carbohydrates, which cause an increase of glucose in the blood, the body will first make them available to all the cells of the body through a hormone called insulin. If there is still a surplus, the body will convert them into fat, and store them in the fat cells for future use.

Without knowing it, we are causing our bodies to accumulate excess fat, yet we are not giving our bodies an opportunity to burn it up. Even if we are not eating excess fat or not converting fat from carbohydrates, we still have an omnivorous diet. This means that we eat at least some fat. If this fat has not been used, it is probably being accumulated in our poor fat cells. Our bodies want to use that fat. So, what is preventing us from using it? We are. We, under the influence of all the propaganda about foods, are imposing this on our bodies. We do it in an innocent way, if you wish.

Our bodies do not want to be carrying around all that fat, plus the water necessary to use it in case of emergency. There is nothing the body can do to stop carrying the water necessary to burn that fat in case it is needed. It is the way it is programmed. But wait—there is someone who can do something about it. That is you! The good news is that every time you let your body burn some of that fat, your body will not have to carry all that surplus water either, and you very quickly lose a few pounds.

Now, you need to know how to give your body the opportunity to rid itself of this extra cargo of water. And this is how: the body normally burns either carbohydrates or fat as a source of energy. But not protein. That is only burned as a source of energy in case there are not enough carbohydrates or fat available, or in case of emergency. It is the essential building block of new cells, for tissue repair, creating antibodies, etc. The key for being able to burn the fat stored in your fat cells is to give your body the opportunity to do it.

The body is always burning energy, even at rest. What is important to know here is that when you eat any kind of carbohydrate, your body will switch from burning stored fat to burning the just-ingested carbohydrates as a source of energy. In essence, you do not need to quit eating carbohydrates—you only need to know *when* to eat carbohydrates, and approximately how long they will prevent you from using your fat stores.

Being aware of what happens in your body when you eat certain foods puts you in control of your weight. For example, if during your meal you have a banana and a glass of orange juice, you know that your body will make those carbohydrates available to all your cells. As soon as your blood glucose goes down to normal levels (which will not take that long), your body will start drawing energy from your fat cells.

A different example is when you eat the kind of complex carbohydrate called starch (like bread, tortillas, and pasta) during your meal. This kind of complex carbohydrate can take up to six hours to be digested. This means that your body will keep absorbing carbohydrates from the digestion of the starch for hours, preventing your body from switching to fat burning. But that is not the only problem. When your body is absorbing the glucose from these carbohydrates, there will be a moment when there is not enough glucose for all the cells of the body, but still the body won't be able to switch to fat burning because of the presence of insulin, and you will feel the strong desire to have something to eat to be able to feed the cells of the body that are practically starving. This normally becomes a vicious cycle that keeps your fat cells full of fat, and unable to burn it off.

We do not understand why many authors writing diet books recommend that people eat complex carbohydrates that are absorbed little by little—they caution fear of the excessive release of insulin. They suggest that this kind of carbohydrate is better for the body, because the insulin released is less. These authors seem to forget that all the cells of the body (except the cells from the brain, liver, and red blood cells) need insulin to be able to use carbohydrates. They seem to forget that while the body is using carbohydrates as a source of energy, it is unable to use its fat stores. And this is one of the main obstacles in anyone's attempt to lose weight.

Also, these authors seem to overlook the fact that insulin is a hormone that, aside from promoting fat storage, also prevents the release of the hormone called glucagon, which is normally the governor in charge of maintaining the level of blood glucose within normal limits. Low blood sugar levels result as a consequence—which is destabilizing for the body. At this point, the body's only recourse is to increase the blood sugar level through the ingestion of carbohydrates. This vicious cycle prevents the body from burning its stores of fat.

TO DRINK OR NOT TO DRINK

If you are used to drinking less water than you actually need, you may have an adaptation process to go through. For one thing, be aware that your body is going to have an abundance of work to do (all that work that has been postponed for years), and you will need to have sufficient rest to make that happen. One other thing—you probably are not used to going to the bathroom frequently. As you begin to drink the water your body needs, you will have to urinate more often, because your bladder won't be used to handling that amount of liquid, and it needs time to recuperate its elasticity. Don't wait until the last moment. Go to the bathroom often at the beginning of the H_2O Diet to prevent any discomfort.

The first phase of the H_2O Diet is to get your body healthier by drinking the water it needs to get the job done, and prepare it for the second phase of the program, where you can eliminate body fat and weight easily. If you suffer from any medical condition like high blood pressure, diabetes, etc., please talk to your doctor about the amount of water you need, and ask for advice on how to increase your intake of water without complications. The first phase will take anywhere from 3 to 6 months. During this phase, you do not have to adapt anything else in your diet, but you have the option to stop eating products made out of ground carbohydrates (i.e., wheat and corn) to reduce the time this phase will take.

While you are on the H_2O Diet, you won't gain volume, even when you keep your normal diet. Just the opposite—you will look slimmer, even if you don't lose weight. And also, be aware that it is possible that your body weight might slightly increase during this phase, because your body's structure will begin to change, becoming more solid. Please be patient, and don't get disappointed with the numbers on your scale. In fact, it would be better if you didn't weigh yourself very often during this phase of the program. Instead, use a measuring tape, and keep a written record of the measurements of your chest, waist, hips, and calves. This will give you a better idea of the effects the H_2O Diet has on your body throughout this process.

The first thing you have to do is an auto analysis of your water-intake habits. Begin by calculating the average amount of water you drink a day. You can include milk, juice and water, but no coffee or sodas containing caffeine, because they are diuretics (i.e., causing you to urinate). If you are drinking less than 6 glasses a day, you will need to increase the amount you drink.

The second element of reorientation is that you have to learn to like water again. If you are not drinking enough water, it is possible that you are in the same situation we were. We had forgotten how to enjoy drinking this most natural of all elements. We would only drink water if there were nothing else on hand. And as you have already read, this is the main source of the problem. Every time we take a sip of soda or eat something sweet between meals, we are preventing our body from doing its normal job. So, it is very important to learn to use our instincts to drink water.

Sipping from drinks is not normal. That is a learned behavior. It is difficult, if not nearly impossible, to drink a complete glass of soda at once. The cold temperature, the gas and the ice make it nearly impossible. Yet it is quite easy to drink a complete glass of water, cool or at room temperature. And the water, instead of altering the state of the body, will actually aid it in performing naturally. It is fine to sip from drinks during meals, or once in a while when drinking your coffee or tea. But it is not okay to be sipping from your coffee or soda all day long. The key here is to learn to drink a full eight-ounce glass of pure water at once. If you have not been drinking enough water, you should start slowly adding more water to your diet. Begin by substituting some of your accustomed drinks after meals for water.

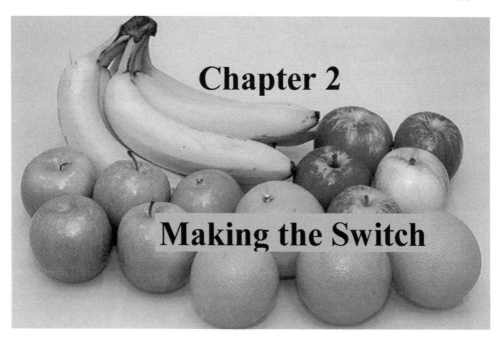

Chapter 2

Making the Switch

BOOSTING YOUR METABOLISM

It takes up to 6 hours to digest foods made out of ground complex carbohydrates like wheat and corn. Unfortunately, having this kind of carbohydrate in your body changes your metabolism. It takes you in a completely different direction than the one you desire. It makes you consume more carbohydrates that are necessary, because the slow release of sugars prevents you from using the fat stored in your fat cells. For some people, once they stop consuming foods containing ground wheat and corn, it takes them up to 2 months to successfully return to their normal selves. But just what is your normal self? If you have never attempted this before, you probably do not know what it feels to be wheat and corn free.

It is a great feeling. A liberation. A sense of control over your own diet and exercise plan with positive results. Actually feeling able to exercise and lose weight, and at the same time enjoying the most delicious foods without the secondary effects of gaining weight. Without this kind of carbohydrate in your body, you won't feel the constant need to snack. And if you do snack, you will be able to go back to fat burning right away. You also will be able to help your body switch to fat burning by light exercising or merely by maintaining an active life style.

If, after reading all this information, you decide to follow the H2O Diet and the strategy to lose weight, we recommend that you take seriously the concept of not consuming wheat and corn products until you reach your goal. Consuming these products at any time during this program would cause a significant delay, and would be very disappointing for you. After you reach your goal, you will be able to consume these products again in moderation as you desire.

After you stop eating wheat and corn products, your metabolism will start changing little by little. The transition could take up to two months. During this process, if you have a craving to snack between meals, you can try to eat fruits, veggies, potato chips, rice cereal with milk, French fries, strawberry shakes (made in the blender with frozen strawberries, milk and sugar), cheesecake (without the crust), rice-flour sugar cookies, or even a milk chocolate bar, etc. This will keep you satisfied, and will not make you gain weight while you are on the H2O Diet. Remember to always read labels and avoid any products that contain wheat, corn, or modified food starch.

You will know that your metabolism has changed (i.e., has become more efficient) when you are able to do your exercise routine at least twice a day on a daily basis. This means that your body is burning the fuels that provide it with energy in a normal manner, which results in improved energy levels.

STEP BY STEP

We need to drink around 6 to 8 eight-ounce glasses of water a day, depending on the activities of the individual. If you exercise or are very active, you will probably have to drink more water than that. Drinks containing caffeine, like coffee and soda, do not count, because they are diuretics (i.e., promote the excretion of urine), and dehydrate your body.

1. The H_2O Diet recommends drinking 1 glass of water when you get up in the morning to recuperate the water lost through evaporation and urine during the night.

2. During your normal breakfast, you should have at least one glass of milk, juice, or water. (You can also drink coffee if you want to, but not as a substitute for the H_2O Diet drink.) Please drink a glass of pure water 45 minutes to 1 hour after breakfast.

3. Drink water as you need between breakfast and lunch. Please try not to drink or eat anything sweet between meals if you can (if you feel you must have a snack, try to eat it at least two hours after your meal).

4. At lunchtime, you can also have the amount of liquids you want with your normal lunch, but drink at least one glass of water, milk, soda, or juice. We also recommend drinking a glass of pure water 45 minutes to 1 hour after every meal to help the body finish its job, and to keep your stomach clean.

5. Drink water as you need between lunch and dinner, depending on the level of activity you have. Again, please try not to drink or eat anything sweet between meals if you

can (but if you must eat something, wait until at least two hours after your meal).

6. Try the same at dinnertime—drink all the liquids you want with your normal dinner, but at least 1 glass of water, milk, soda, or juice. And don't forget to drink your glass of water 45 minutes to 1 hour after your meal.

7. We also recommend drinking a glass of water before going to bed, depending, of course, on how long ago you drank your last glass of water.

8. You can drink more or less water than is recommended here, depending on your individual activities.

STARCHES AND THE H2O DIET

The first phase of our H2O Diet is to focus on smart water consumption. The second phase is to switch from burning carbohydrates to burning fat reserves. We really encourage you to carefully read this section on the process of switching over. When you understand how your body switches from using carbohydrates to using fats as a source of energy, you will be home free.

Due to the fact that we are omnivorous, we can obtain energy from different sources. Our body is adapted to obtain energy from carbohydrates, fat, and also protein. When you have a combination of these three sources in your meal, there is a strict order in which these nutrients will be used as a source of energy: carbohydrates will be used first, fat second, and protein will be used only in case of emergency, when we are lacking sufficient carbohydrates and fats.

Here we are only going to talk about the way our body uses the fat and carbohydrates in our diet. Normally, a well-balanced meal will contain: simple and complex carbohydrates, fat, protein, and water, as well as numerous minerals and vitamins. And this is how it unfolds. Let's say you had an apple, a slice of bread, an egg, and a glass of milk for breakfast. This meal contains the three macronutrients that we need to obtain energy. The apple contains simple carbohydrates that will be converted to simple sugars and absorbed by the small intestine into the bloodstream. These sugars will be transported to the liver to be converted into glucose. At the moment the blood sugar rises, the insulin hormone will be released from the beta cells in the pancreas into the blood stream.

Insulin helps control the amount of sugar in the blood, and makes glucose available to most of the cells in the body (the brain and the liver do not need insulin to be able to absorb glucose). At the same time, insulin promotes the storage of fats in the fat cells. This is very important to understand. Every time you eat a carbohydrate (i.e., sugar in the form of candy, pastry, bread, drinks containing sugar, etc.), the immediate response of the body is the release of insulin, regardless of the amount of sugar. The effect is the same: at that time, you automatically switch to burning carbohydrates instead of fat as a source of energy.

If the amount of carbohydrates consumed is more than the amount the body can store in the liver and muscles (there is a very limited amount of carbohydrates that the body actually can store), the extra carbohydrates will be converted to fat, and held in reserve in the fat cells. Always remember that every time you take a sip of soda or eat a piece of candy or a slice of bread, you will be switching from burning fat to burning carbohydrates as a source of energy. It is like trying to keep your fireplace burning with paper and cardboard—you would have to be constantly feeding your fire to keep the flame going.

The problem is *not* that carbohydrates are a bad source of energy. Just the opposite: they are an excellent source of energy when used properly. The problems begin if you depend on your energy from carbohydrates most of the time. You need to give your body a break. You need to let your body use the fat that has been stored everywhere over your body for years. Being omnivorous means we eat all kinds of things, including fat. And the only way for our body to use the fats stored in our fat cells is to stop producing insulin all day long. This does not mean that you have to stop eating carbohydrates. This means that you should eat a well-balanced meal at mealtime, including your dessert.

Your body will use the food as a source of energy in the same order all the time. First, the body will use the simple carbohydrates, then the complex carbohydrates, because they take longer to digest. The fats have to go through an even more complex process before they can be used as a source of energy. Something very important to remember: fats cannot be used as a source of energy in the presence of insulin. Insulin promotes the storage of fat.

We are gaining weight because we have the wrong formula. Eating is an immense job for the body. It takes a great amount of energy to process the food we eat. When we eat more that we need, we are burdening our bodies. We probably feel exhausted, and in need of rest. Thus begins a vicious cycle. And because we are tired, we don't feel like exercising.

GIVE YOUR BODY A BREAK

Are starches preventing you from switching over? Because starches are complex carbohydrates (chains of sugars), they take longer to digest. With an absorption rate of two calories per minute, it could take up to 6 hours for starches to get digested. All this time, depending on the amount of sugar being released from the starches, insulin is continually being secreted into the bloodstream to lower the blood-glucose level. This constant release of insulin prevents the body from switching from using carbohydrates as a source of energy, to using fats.

After some time, the amount of sugars being absorbed by the small intestine into the bloodstream from the complex carbohydrates is no longer enough to feed all the cells, but is enough to cause the release of insulin (preventing you from using the fat stored in your fat cells). In a short amount of time, you will feel hungry for fuel you can use immediately as a source of energy—simple carbohydrates (and the cycle begins again).

How can you switch from getting energy mostly from carbohydrates to getting energy from the fat you have stored in your fat cells? The first thing you have to do is to try to understand the concept of how carbohydrates and fats are used as sources of energy. If you have doubts after the following explanation, ask your doctor specific questions, or investigate in nutrition books and online. The second thing is to do an analysis of your water-intake habits, and follow the H2O Diet in an attempt to get your body into a perfect equilibrium.

The human body really loves carbohydrates (in the form of glucose)—especially the brain. In fact, glucose is the only source of energy that the brain uses, and it needs no insulin to absorb it. We could live happy with just a minimum amount of glucose for the use of the brain, to use during digestion by all the cells of the body, and during fat breakdown. Also, the body has a limited capacity to store glucose. The excess is converted to fat and stored in the fat cells.

In a normal diet, after completion of digestion, the body should switch to burning fat as a source of energy. Only the brain and the liver keep using glucose from reserves. Also, the stored glucose can be used in case of emergency by all the cells of the body when the person is in danger and releases the adrenaline hormone. The other problem is that the fat produced from excess carbohydrate intake is formed by non-essential fatty acids. That means that the body will give preference to fatty acids that are provided by the diet, and that are essential. When the reserves of glucose go down, the body makes you feel hungry. Remember that the body has the capacity to store enough glucose to last from 8-12 hours, so you should not be hungry 1 hour after you just ate, unless you are in a vicious cycle, and are having trouble switching to fat burning.

The third element that really helps to switch to fat burning is to control the amount of products made out of ground complex carbohydrates in the diet—like bread, pasta, cereals, and tortillas made from wheat and corn, that take up to 6 hours to digest. Substitute instead carbohydrates like carrots, celery, tomatoes, lettuce, fruits, beans, rice, potatoes, nuts, etc., that the body burns faster. Ground complex carbohydrates are loaded with chains of sugars, and take much longer to digest. And because they are ground, and also contain little fiber, they will be absorbed almost completely in the small intestine.

All these carbohydrates are more than the body normally needs, and the extra amount consumed will be converted to fat. If you substitute this variety of complex carbohydrates (i.e., wheat and corn) by eating vegetables like carrots and tomatoes and fruits, beans, rice, potatoes, and so on, during your intent to switch, your body will use them right away, and will also replenish the stored reserves. In this way, you would save your body the effort of converting carbohydrates to fat. You will also discover that you can eat your normal meal, even a dessert (with exception of products made out of wheat and corn), and that you will not feel hungry right away. But don't forget to stick to the H2O Diet during this entire process.

It is very important to try to maintain a perfect equilibrium in your body. Also, with the fat provided by your normal diet and the fat stored in the fat cells, you should not have any problems. Remember, the only thing you are going to substitute is fresh fruits and vegetables, in place of ground complex carbohydrates. Potatoes and rice can still be included in your diet, because they are burned faster than corn and wheat.

ELIMINATE THE SURPLUS SALT

The body strives for an equilibrium in the amount of liquids it contains. Salt, potassium, and calcium are very important in regulating the amount of liquids in your system. Any change in the concentration of salt and potassium causes a switch between the intracellular and extracellular fluids. When you start drinking the water your body needs, it is possible that your body will need to get rid of some salt. This is because it will not need to retain extra water.

When you don't drink enough water, the body starts retaining some water and recycling it. To do this, it needs salt. There are several ways for the body to eliminate the accumulated salt. Normally, you eliminate salt through sweat and urine. Ingesting foods containing calcium, like milk, can also accelerate the elimination of salt by the kidneys and the salivary glands. Another way to accelerate the elimination of the extra salt is by eating products rich in potassium, like bananas, watermelon, melon, apples, orange juice, etc.

FATS FROM CARBOHYDRATES

Did you know that the human body is capable of making fat out of carbohydrates like bread, tortillas, pasta, etc.? As we explained previously, we have a restricted capacity to store carbohydrates in our body. Most people do not know what happens when we eat excess carbohydrates. Those excess carbohydrates in our diet get converted to fat. It is not easy for the body to perform this task. It literally takes the energy out of you. It is a strenuous job. And why?

Why does our body even have to make fat? That's precisely the problem. We do not have to do that. It's like needlessly working overtime. Our normal diet contains all the fat we need. Our bodies do not need to produce all that extra fat. That is one of the reasons why some people have been overweight, even while being extra careful not to eat excess fatty foods. The problem is not only producing the fat. It is a chain of events. All the extra effort to produce this fat makes your body tired, and you become more sedentary.

Products made out of complex carbohydrates that are ground—like bread, tortillas, and pasta—are slowly, but almost completely, absorbed by the body in the small intestine. This kind of food provides the body with more carbohydrates than can be stored as glycogen. Also, the slow release of glucose from this kind of carbohydrate prevents the body from using the fats stored in the body, for a longer time than simple carbohydrates do. That's one of the reasons why people feel hungry, even when they have just eaten.

When the glucose released from these carbohydrates is not enough to feed all the cells of the body, but is enough to raise the glucose in the bloodstream to stimulate the production of insulin by the pancreas, we enter into a vicious cycle that prevents the body from using fat as a source of energy. At that moment, when the body is prevented by the circulating insulin from using the fat stored in the fat cells, you will be feeling the strong sensation of needing something to eat.

Let's see what happens when you eat a complete meal. Following a meal including protein, fat, complex carbohydrates, simple carbohydrates, vitamins, and minerals, the body releases insulin. Glucose flows to all the cells in the body. Unfortunately, the body is unable to use the stored fats in the presence of insulin, but is very happy with the glucose. Carbohydrates get stored as glycogen, mainly for the use of the brain when insulin is not present. Fat is stored in the fat cells. Excess carbohydrates get converted to fat.

Complex carbohydrates are absorbed in the small intestine and converted to glucose, slowly rising the blood glucose level. Insulin continues being released to lower glucose levels in the blood, and to make the glucose available to cells. Not enough glucose is circulating in the bloodstream for the needs of all the cells of the body, but the body is unable to use fat in the presence of insulin. The individual feels pangs of hunger for sweets (simple carbohydrates that are an inmediate source of energy). He or she responds by snacking, and the cycle starts again.

Carbohydrates are a treat for the body, but can also become a nightmare. After researching all the information about the way our body digests the carbohydrates and fats from our diet, the conclusions are the following: no one who is overweight should be eating on a regular basis any kind of products made out of complex carbohydrates that are ground, like wheat, corn, etc., while trying to lose the fat accumulated in their bodies throughout years. When you begin the second phase of the H2O Diet, immediately stop your intake of bread, pasta, cereals, tortillas, etc., made out of wheat and corn.

Exercise lightly to help your body switch from using carbohydrates as a source of energy, to using fat. Once you are in the second phase of the H2O Diet, after you have stopped eating wheat and corn products, your body will easily be able to make that switch. We saw that just after you eat, simple carbohydrates are used first as a source of energy. A way to help your body to switch is by doing a little exercise. This does not have to be formal exercise. Walking, taking the stairs at work instead of the elevator, or two minutes of simple stretching exercises would do it.

To lose weight, just as to win a chess game, you have to have a strategy. A good diet plan is similar to playing a chess game successfully—to win the game or to lose weight, you have to look ahead several steps, and evaluate every possibility before you make a move. Adjust your favorite meals to the program and follow the recommendations to lose weight permanently. Be aware that giving in on some foods that are not allowed would send you back to the beginning of the program again. This is because these foods would change your metabolism back (making it less efficient), and it could take you up to two months to get back to where you were.

The signs and symptoms that tell you that your metabolism is not working as it should be, are the following: binge eating, tiredness, no desire to exercise, and the impossibility of switching to fat burning because of the amount of carbohydrates consumed. The good news is that after you reach your target weight, you will be able to eat—on your own terms—the foods that are not allowed while you are in the process of losing weight. Just keep an eye on your weight, and don't let these foods take control of your life. So, be creative with your diet—the limit is your imagination. There are plenty of delicious foods to enjoy while you are on the H2O Diet.

A diet consists of everything a person eats. What makes a good diet is the nutritious content, the variety of nutrients available, and the adjustment of the diet to the personal needs, according to many factors like age, environmental changes, physical activity, illnesses, etc.

NUTRITIONAL NEEDS

In general, the focus of every meal is to include some of each group of the following nutrients in a variety of foods:

Proteins (Examples: steak, pork, chicken, fish, eggs, milk, shrimp, beans, nuts, soy, etc.).

Fats (Examples: butter, bacon, olive oil, soy bean oil, fat contained in meat and other foods).

Carbohydrates (Examples: sugar, fruits, fruit juice, vegetables, grains and cereals, etc.).

Vitamins (Examples: vitamin A, vitamin C—found in many fruits and vegetables, and vitamin D—produced by the body's exposure to sunlight; also found in enriched milk).

Minerals (Examples: calcium—found in milk, cheese, and broccoli; potassium—found in orange juice, bananas, melon and watermelon).

Note: Vitamin D, resulting from at least a 5-minute daily exposure to the sun, is essential for absorbing calcium.

All foods need to be consumed in moderation. Too much of the same thing can become unhealthy. Even drinking water can be fatal for someone who drinks H2O to excess (water poisoning). Eating reasonable portions of a variety of foods is the best way of obtaining the different nutriments needed for optimal health. Foods should always be chosen while taking into consideration the nutritional needs and preferences of the individual.

EXERCISE

Exercise is a must for everyday life in order to maintain strength and health. The following is an easy, doable, cheap, and effective exercise plan to help people lose weight. The only equipment needed is a pair of dumbbells (5-pound, or 10-pound will do). From the beginning, keep a running record of your measurements: chest, waist, hips, thighs, and calves.

For losing weight permanently, the best time to exercise is when your body is using fat as a source of energy. This time is when you are not burning carbohydrates as a source of energy. Exercising at least 2 hours after a meal, up to 1 hour before a meal, will burn the most fat. The ideal time is in the morning, right after getting up and drinking some water to hydrate, and before taking a shower. At this time, you are for sure getting energy from fat. Also, exercise while watching your favorite program or the news—3 to 5 minutes at a time is sufficient. Then take a break and do it again. Exercising is not recommended right before or right after a meal, because it has been shown to cause health problems. Talk to your doctor before starting any kind of diet or exercise program.

Any time is the perfect time to start with this exercise plan. Start slowly, at your own pace, with the easiest exercises. The more exercise you do, the easier it will be the next time. Exercise 3 to 5 minutes at a time, for 2 to 6 times a day, or more if you feel in the mood. Some days you may exercise only 2 times, or none at all if you are not feeling well, and that is okay. Only exercise when you feel comfortable doing it. You are in this for the long run.

EXERCISE ROUTINES

Do only the exercises that seem easy for you to do. You may add some more later to your routine as you feel fit. You can repeat each of the exercises as many times as you want. Changing from one exercise to another allows your muscles to recuperate, and lets you vary from one to another until you are done exercising.

Swimming in the Air is the best exercise to move the majority of the muscles of the body. It somehow mimics swimming backwards in the water. Move your arms at the same time that you flex your legs, and tilt your head slightly down to the front. This is an easy exercise that warms you up for the other ones in the routine.
Start with: 5-10 repetitions at a time. Goal: 40 at a time.

Knee-Bends are the most difficult exercise in this routine, and are not recommended for people with knee problems, or other health problems. They quickly increase the strength in your legs. This is the most effective exercise to cause you to burn fat. You can feel how they warm you up right away. Start slowly and carefully. Stand erect. Keeping your eyes on the horizon and your back straight, lower your body simply by bending your knees. At the beginning, you can use your hands to help you support your weight, until you get enough resistance to do it as you wish. As you do the knee-bends, put

your hands over your thighs, and slide them down just above your knees, then push yourself up.
Start with: 3 to 5 repetitions at a time. Goal: 10-15 at a time.

Swinging Arms gives you time to relax your legs while you swing your bent arms in a rowing motion back and forth horizontally. Start out by standing straight, then move your arms, and at the same time, contract the muscles of your shoulders, and turn your head slightly to the left and to the right. Not only does it loosen up your shoulders and arms, but also gives you time to relax your legs, and gets you ready for the next exercise where you exercise your legs again.
Start with: 5-10 repetitions at a time. Goal: 40 at a time.

High-Rise Leg-Ups is an excellent exercise to give you sufficient resistance to start using the stairs instead of the elevator, and also more resistance for walking. Standing, lift a leg with bent knee until the thigh is horizontal, then repeat with the opposite leg.
Start with: 5-10 repetitions at a time. Goal: 40 at a time.

Bend-Overs are great for the face. Just start standing straight with feet spread slightly apart, then bending over several times. You can do whatever you want with your arms and hands at the same time, like extending them and trying to touch the floor, or just keeping them planted on your hips.
Start with: 5-10 repetitions at a time. Goal: 40 at a time.

Stretching. After doing a few exercises, and at the end of your routine, you should try to relax your muscles by doing some stretching. Pull your arms up over your head, and hold one of your hands with the other one. Move your hands together sideways to stretch your muscles from your back.
Start with: 5-10 repetitions at a time. Goal: 40 at a time.

Lifting Weights (5-10 pound dumbbells). This exercise should be started a few days after the beginning of the exercise program to give you ample time to build up some endurance. Once you are ready to do weights, start little by little with a variety of lifts with the 5-pound dumbbells. Move up to the 10-pound dumbbells whenever you feel ready to do so.
Start with: 5-10 repetitions at a time. Goal: open-ended.

EXERCISE AND THE ELECTROLYTE BALANCE

Some water is stored away in the body as a proportion of the reserves of fat and carbohydrates. This proportion is related to the amount of water the body needs in order to burn calories from fat and carbohydrates. Exercise burns calories from fat and carbohydrates and releases water. When you exercise and consequently burn fat and carbohydrates, your body releases the water that has been stored for this purpose.

After you exercise, make sure you include in your diet the foods that contain the necessary electrolytes (i.e., potassium and calcium) to eliminate the extra water circulating in your body, to prevent your body from restoring the fat you have burned. You only have to deal with the water released from burning fat. The water stored for carbohydrates always remains basically the same amount. In the exercise section, we explain when to exercise to make sure you are burning fat to lose weight.

Once you start your exercise routine and you include in your daily diet foods rich in calcium and potassium, you will start losing weight in about a week or a week and a half. This is because your body needs to get used to the exercise routine, and sometimes it has to retain some liquids to be able to repair the initial damage caused to the tissues by the exercise. At this point, we recommend that you weigh yourself twice a day, morning and night, and record your weight daily in a log.

Be aware that when you become ill, you often gain weight, due to the body's tendency to retain water to combat the illness. If that is the case, you can lose this unwelcome weight soon after you recover—if you continue following this program, and keep the faith that you can do it.

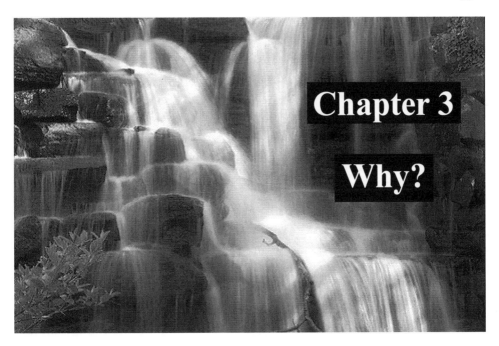

Chapter 3

Why?

SIMPLIFY

We are talking about a simple, painless route to happiness, not the agonizing roller coaster of self-denial followed by disillusionment. As is often the case, the simplest strategy to resolve complex problems yields the truest solution. This guidebook will present the reader with a practical, painless, logical approach for achieving physical and mental harmony. The H_2O Diet does not involve any extraordinary sacrifice, suffering, or unwarranted discipline. Most diets, if not all, claim to help you shed pounds and attain your ideal self, yet are doomed to failure. They are basically contrary to human nature. Our approach conforms to reality. It is a natural path to achieving health by consuming water—something your doctor has probably recommended many times, and one that remains the most-amazing medicine, one that is available without prescription or exorbitant cost.

How strange that when you listen to your doctor recommend drinking up to 8 glasses of water a day, it seems preposterous. Why would he propose such a regime? As he moves on to other observations and recommendations, his suggestion is lost in the muddle of information. It was never properly focused on, and never adequately explained in the context of *your* life. Besides, you suffer no obvious dehydration nor side effects from lack of that vital fluid. You might consume too much coffee, soda, and beer, but those liquids are more than enough in themselves to keep you afloat.

CAFFEINE ADDICTION

Paul is an acquaintance. He was a wreck. He knew he was consuming too much caffeine in his coffee and sodas, yet clung to his belief that a liquid is a liquid. His morning began with his ritual coffee and the morning paper. During the day when he was thirsty and needed a lift, he drank an ice-cold cola, then another, then another. He was subconsciously swayed by the persistent advertising of his favorite caffeine drinks, and seemed to not only quench his thirst with them, but also received a dose of energy that kept him on target.

Paul was a habitual consumer of a stimulant that triggered his heart and central nervous system to artificial hyperactivity. No wonder he was drained by the end of the day. His sleep was intermittent and troubled. He developed dark circles under his eyes, which he attributed to his hectic job and the worries that rattled around inside his head 24 hours a day. Paul was burned out, yet he had no idea much of it was self-induced and easily preventable.

When Paul first heard of our theories that an intelligent, systematic consumption of water could alter his addictive behavior and thus break his caffeine cycle, he was dubious. As the logic of our approach began to soak in, he decided to see for himself if it really worked. The first step was to realize that the most natural nutriment for the human body is water. The next step was to begin to drink a glass of water to supplement his intake of coffee and sodas, then to quench the phantom hunger that plagued him between meals.

He discovered his body eliminating wastes in a natural fashion, stimulating a sounder appetite, reducing a good degree of mental and physical fatigue, draining the excess fat from his face and body, and giving him a new outlook on life. What did it cost him? Very little: just the small amount of discipline to drink a glass of water according to a simple plan. He became a new person with just a few common-sense adaptations to his normal regimen. He drained his body of poisons, and did not replace them—because he did not have the cravings to do so. Is it possible that drinking a glass of water can break the chain of addiction? Just try it.

H2O

H_2O is an innocuous little molecule that comprises the oceans and streams that cover the earth, the ice at the North and South Poles, the ice in our ice-cube trays, as well as the clouds in the heavens, and the air we breathe. It is a clear, colorless, odorless and tasteless liquid, essential for most plant and animal life. Water is a family of 2 hydrogen atoms bound together with an oxygen atom to form a bipolar molecule that acts as a slippery magnet. It also comprises some two-thirds of our bodies, where the natural properties of water allow it to dissolve a variety of substances, and transport them to the 100 trillion cells that depend on the sustenance and oxygen it carries. The water-based plasma also transports hormones, antibodies, red blood cells, nutriments, etc. in the blood stream to the cells. The cells, in turn, exchange waste materials and CO_2 to be carried away, filtered, and expelled from the body principally as urine, perspiration, tears, and breath. Think of each group of cells as a town on a river, dependent on the river for drinking water, nutrients, bathing, irrigation, transportation, recreation, and sewage disposal. Deprive the body of sufficient amounts of this remarkable molecule, and it withers and dies like a field of corn in a drought.

CHANGES

Saturate the blood with alcohol, caffeine, excess sugars, and who knows what else, and the body diverts its focus to neutralizing and eliminating these foreign bodies. Excess sugar = excess fat. What does your cornfield do when acid rain pours down on it, insecticides leach into its roots, and its air is befouled with smog? It gets a little weak—insects and fungi find it an easy target to invade, and its ears of corn shrink.

Listen to your body, tune in to its ills, and focus on its needs. Once you begin to substitute H_2O for the poisons and refuse to ingest them, you begin to reverse the damage. Harmful, useless and excess chemicals are flushed from your cells. Your body will now have sufficient water to metabolize, repair, and otherwise function properly, and even an excess amount of water to accomplish the tasks lowest on its hierarchy of survival priorities.

As your body requests healthier, essential food elements, your positive response allows your mind to achieve a higher mental state, your physical energies to increase, dry skin and pimples to clear up, organs to work less—the whole organism begins more to resemble its optimal form. Excess fat is diminished without the pain of a forced, unnatural diet. You become a new you, and on a permanent basis. Fatigue, vagueness, high blood pressure, excess salt and its effects are all diminished. Ask your doctor if water alone is not a reasonable, sound beginning to creating a healthier human being. Prove us wrong. Drink water according to our recommendations, and observe and feel the results. What do you have to lose?

Do not focus on the weight that pops up on your scale. The object of this diet is not to "diet" so much as it is to create the right conditions for your body to demand its proper nutrition. You automatically will lose weight in the right places, lose puffiness that bloats your face, waist and thighs— yet that metamorphosis is a secondary effect. The principal goal of the H2O Diet is simply to feel better. It is a question of quality vs. quantity.

Your focus should be on regaining vitality and appearance by doing something that is most natural to your well-being: consuming enough water for your body to function properly. As you do so, expect your complexion to adapt to a sufficient water supply. Your skin will become less oily as the waste products are flushed out; your color will change to a healthier hue; your dry, wrinkled skin will assume a new, more youthful texture. Slowly, your mental faculties will sharpen; you will feel an infusion of "get up and go." These will not be dramatic, immediate results, but will gradually build as your body and mind adapt to your new state of being.

You should also feel the need to exercise. It is one of the fundamental elements of the human character, and should remain in tune with your instincts. Do not attempt to leap tall buildings at a single bound. Respond to your body's need by taking a walk or going for a swim. Do something enjoyable to recapture the elasticity and resistance of youth. You should not imagine that you can spin time backward, but rather should set realistic goals and expectations. Focus on the pleasure of a habitual activity. Walk, trot or run, yet take time to enjoy your surroundings: the deep blue of the sky, the shades of green, the flowers, birds, sidewalks and buildings that inhabit your world. Diets tend to be born of desperation and idealistic expectations, yet die in the cold reality of unrelenting pain and depredation. Always think positively, and treat yourself with respect. Drink a little water; eat sensibly, but as you wish; listen to your self and act on your particular desires; enjoy life as your world begins to fall into place. Perhaps water *is* the elixir of life.

SOUND FOOD

Common sense tells you what to eat. Once a good deal of the phantom cravings due to lack of water are subverted, subtle appetites are aroused. Instead of dipping your hand into a bag of junk food, you might listen to your inner voice suggest a nectarine or an orange. That cup of coffee in the morning is delicious and stimulating, yet is also a diuretic (i.e., a substance that increases the excretion of urine). Many sodas are also diuretics. Instead of satisfying your thirst, they give the illusion of liquefying the body, yet actually deprive it of its water supply.

Knowing this, it is a simple procedure to drink a glass of water soon after that morning coffee, or even substitute those cups of coffee and sodas with water. Doing the latter, you avoid introducing sugars, stimulants, dyes and gases that occupy your body's digestive system with a formidable cleansing task. Instead, consuming pure water allows the body to correctly seek its own homeostasis—to balance itself as it performs countless biochemical and physiological chores.

Many dieticians would tell you how to eat a well-rounded diet. They assert that the majority of your food should consist of grains: bread, pasta, crackers, cereal, rolls, pancakes, etc. Beware! Instead, focus on trying to eat 3 to 5 servings of vegetables a day: carrots, broccoli, cauliflower, lettuce, tomatoes, potatoes, etc. Also, keep fruits on hand. Try to eat 2 to 4 servings a day of: apples, oranges, peaches, grapes, bananas, kiwi fruit, strawberries, melons, etc. Meat, fish, poultry and eggs are important to a well-rounded diet, but 2 to 3 servings a day are sufficient. The same number of servings is indicated for dairy products: milk, cheese, yogurt, ice cream, etc. Fats, oils and sweets are to be used sparingly. You are what you eat. If you are to enjoy the benefits of good health, a little common sense is not much to ask of yourself. Good sense can become habitual.

HYDRATE

It seems that when the body is in a state of dehydration, the solution would be simple enough: ingest any liquid and saturate the body with water. Not so. Imagine a dehydrated plum—a prune. Soak it with water, and it fails to become a plum again. Although substances like powdered milk can resume something close to their former states by being dissolved in water, the human body is much more complex. It is more like trying to hydrate a dried rose. Even if you begin to administer an adequate supply of water to a withered rose before it becomes dried out, it takes time for it to recover. The human body is involved in such a multiplicity of labors, that once water has been drained from the system, it takes a concerted effort for the body to assimilate fluid and regenerate its functions to a satisfactory level.

As the body loses water, it prioritizes the use it puts the little remaining water to. Certain systems must be shut down, others must work on a limited budget of water, while still others remain vital. The body goes into shock. Salts and uric acids pile up, sweating is reduced, housecleaning is put on hold, crisis management insists on lower energy levels—the body switches to a survival mode. As soon as water is reintroduced in sufficient amounts into the system, recovery begins by gearing up the sewage system: salts and unsavory acids are washed away; cell wastes flow into the bloodstream to be filtered out by the kidneys; healing accelerates. Enzymes (the organic catalysts in our bodies) begin to be churned out to aid in regenerating and revitalizing the body; hormones (chemical messengers produced by endocrine glands) stream out of the adrenal, pituitary, thyroid, parathyroid, pancreas, ovary, placenta and testis. Lethargy begins to melt away. The body begins to awaken from a self-induced stupor.

GET REAL

The mind, although a miraculous creation, exists on a multiplicity of fragile, interdependent levels. Instincts are often dominated, even ignored by the intellect. Even survival is often subverted to the impulses for love, bravery, honor, or pure illusion. The vogue for the ideal shape also can lead us down a precarious path. While the true nature of our selves is screaming out for sound nourishment, we punish our appetites with self-denial and foolish substitutes. That perfect exterior is probably at best a figment of our imaginations. Why not instead seek beauty in balance, happiness in self-fulfillment? Just as our actions trigger an endless echo of reactions and counter actions, so do our heedless pursuits of detrimental diets, junk food parfaits, and mindless credence. Go back to the basics. Keep it simple.

Money. In our modern society, we tend to make fancy formulas to equate all human endeavors to dollars. Happily, your venture into the H_2O Diet should probably prove to be a cost-efficient effort. Consider this workbook as your guideline, your coach, and equate its cost to that of a professional doing the same job. How much would it cost you to contract a personal trainer at a health spa or a fitness center? In one hour's time your workbook will have paid for itself—yet it is there for you to consult day and night at your slightest whim. How much does its main component cost? Tap water is virtually free, bottled water at a supermarket costs about 50 cents for a 12-ounce bottle, or a dollar for a gallon container. You do not have to run to your doctor, then your pharmacy, for a prescription and refills. When you are away from home, you have easy access to your diet supplement. What could be more natural than an occasional drink of water?

What is it worth to clear your medicine cabinet of half the medications that decay on the shelves? What is the price of a mind that is no longer gummed up with useless chemicals? Dust it out like an abandoned attic—rediscover the treasures that patiently lie awaiting liberation. Have you noticed how your car runs after a tune up? Your body is probably also way past due for a tune up. How much would you pay for the taste of a fresh apple or strawberry? What is the true worth of a sense of well-being and purpose?

Keep on eating the foods you currently do. Enjoy the occasional excesses, but keep focused on common sense. After each binge on some forbidden fruit, toast yourself with a glass of water. As your body flushes itself of toxins and begins to recuperate its normal functions, listen to it. If you have a craving for fruits and vegetables, satisfy that inner voice. Tune in to yourself. If you have an insistent craving for sweets or junk food or something saturated with fats, attempt to satisfy that impulse with a glass of water. Then give in without guilt when you must. But do not lose your edge.

This is not a battle of will; it is more a conditioning to a new approach of fulfilling your appetites. Change your attitude: treat that glass of water as if it were fresh from an icy mountain stream. If it is warm, imagine it to be a soothing cup of Indonesian tea. Do not drown your garden; simply give it the water it needs to thrive and blossom. Drink with enthusiasm, knowing it is the essence of what your body truly desires.

At the onset of these essential changes, your body will be working hard to reorient itself. Take time to rest and permit your body to do its job adequately. Normal activity should be sufficient to stimulate your system to detoxify itself. Once you feel yourself over the initial impact of taking in a sufficient water supply, you should feel inclined to become more active. Most of all, stay within the bounds of what is reasonable for you yourself.

Do not try to achieve levels of physical activity meant for someone else. If you wish to be less sedentary, schedule a daily walk. If you are already active and feel in need of greater activity, play tennis, golf, or some other sport that pleases you. If you attempt to force yourself into a role that does not fit you well, you are inviting failure. Begin the chain of success by being reasonable, and developing a dialogue with your own personal needs and desires.

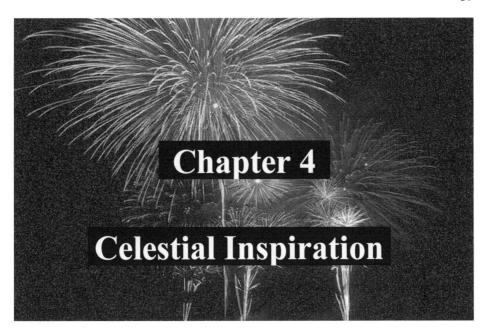

Chapter 4

Celestial Inspiration

We neither condone nor refute any religious beliefs. That said, we might make mention of a historical/religious figure for his insightful philosophy, and attempt to put it to use in our focus on the interplay of health, diet and well-being. Indeed, one of our major expected outcomes of our new awareness is to regain control of our own lives. It is based on the amazing potential a simple glass of water holds.

BUDDHA

In 566 B.C. Siddhartha Gautama (i.e., Buddha—"the Enlightened One") was born to a local ruler of a kingdom stretching out on the western slopes of the Himalaya. Being raised in luxury, Buddha married at the tender age of 16, as was the custom of his times and rank. Subsequently, Siddhartha led a life of royal ease in his father's palace, leaving his sanctuary only 4 times. On those brief sojourns, he met up with an old man, a sick man, a dead man, and a religious man. He became burdened with his discovery, and rationalized that man's existence on earth is bordered by the ultimate finality of sickness, old age, and death. On his 29th birthday, he escaped the palace and fled to the edge of a forest where he cut his hair and shed the royal trappings he wore, exchanging them for the tattered clothing of a hunter he befriended. Thus began his wanderings. During this period of self-denial, he studied a variety of religious beliefs, leading the contemplative life of an ascetic.

Just like Siddhartha, we have all been down the path of self-discovery. In youth we enjoy the luxury of a healthy, fit body, and a spirit that knows no bounds. As we pass through adolescence and adulthood, we encounter dramatic changes in our philosophy: new ideas surge to replace worn-out ones that soon fade into the past, barely leaving an echo. We seek to recapture the vitality and fitness of our youth by investigating and experimenting with new methods of nutrition and awareness.

In our constant testing of theories to capture that shadowy ideal of ourselves, concepts that we discover to be perverted and erroneous are confronted by new evidence, and left behind. We attain new beliefs by gradually stripping away ones we consider to be false. Our way of talking, dressing, acting—even believing—changes. We seek a true balance of body and spirit through one diet after another, one worldview after another, discarding beliefs as they prove unobtainable or too painful.

Finally, in 531 B.C., made aware of his approaching awakening by a vivid dream, he sat beneath a pipal tree (i.e., the bo tree—an Indian fig tree), where he began to meditate on the meaning of this earthly existence. After a period of intense meditation and abstinence, the Four Noble Truths were revealed to him: (1) this existence consists of suffering; (2) this suffering has a cause; (3) that cause can be brought to an end; (4) one must exhibit the necessary discipline to bring it to an end. Once 7 days had passed on his throne of awakening, Siddhartha moved to the other side of the pipal tree and remained there meditating and fasting for an additional 5 weeks. He then walked to Lake Muchalinda where he was deluged in a 7-day rain.

We have all had dreams of our ideal selves. We have meditated in the bosom of our homes, and then launched ourselves on a metaphysical journey to attain that ideal self. After a considerable period of self-denial and near starvation, we realize that dieting is essentially suffering. Our suffering is unnatural and insupportable; it therefore must come to an end. There must be a discipline that is more natural and less intrusive. Our salvation begins when we initiate a water diet, and find a solution so natural and so direct, it is a true revelation.

Later, returning to the pipal tree, he considered preaching his newfound truths to the world, yet feared that his profound verities were beyond the capacity for most men to understand. He thought of human beings like lotuses, many blooming on the surface of the water, some submerged deep below the surface, and some nearly ready to emerge. He decided to attempt to reach those about to emerge. Thus began his 45-year public ministry.

This H2O Diet is ingeniously, deceivingly simple. You can tell your friends about it, but too many are immersed in the beliefs of the false idols that plague our society: a bombardment of advertising that stimulates our appetites to consume wholesale amounts snacks, sodas, and fats. On the other hand, many are discovering the simple joys of eating to supplement the basic body needs. And some are ready to discover the easy, natural path to recovery—a glass of water.

THE PATH TO HAPPINESS

Siddhartha discovered his Noble Eightfold Path to achieve true happiness: (1) right speech exhibits itself in refraining from vulgarities, lies, and malicious, abusive speech; (2) right conduct entails not killing nor stealing, and remaining chaste; (3) right livelihood signifies earning a living in an honest way, as well as practicing friendship, compassion, sympathetic joy, and an evenness of temper; (4) right effort requires a conscious attempt to employ correct strategies to reach a goal; (5) right mindfulness is achieved by refusing to be taken in by superficial sensual pleasures and material possessions, but rather by filling the mind with uplifting energy; (6) right concentration implies blocking out extraneous interferences to achieve valid outcomes; (7) right views implies focusing on the world as it really is, by not mistaking the impermanent for the permanent, the unpleasant for the pleasant; (8) right intentions allow one to avoid the pitfalls of energies misdirected on false desires.

Our ultimate goal is the happiness realized by freeing ourselves from the frustration and suffering brought about by our present state of body and mind. To do so, we may choose to follow a path similar to Siddhartha's 8 steps: (1) Refrain from deceiving language; neither accept it from outside sources, nor generate it from within. Do not let the invasive voice of advertising introduce deceitful appetites, nor trigger your response to purchase and consume their products. (2) Be gentle, especially with yourself. Respect your personal needs, yet let water help curb them to fit the realities of your true desires. There is no need for self-induced punishment, nor a killing of your desires; simply reshape and redirect them. (3) Friendship, compassion, joy, and an even temper come automatically when you are feeling good. The chain reaction begins with abundant water, then leads to a slimmer appearance, better bodily functions, a fresh outlook—a painless recovery that evokes the positive emotions which make you feel alive, and attractive to others. (4) Focus your effort on our techniques to launch you on a new path. Adapt them to fit you and your lifestyle. (5) From your determination to make the slight changes which result in huge modifications in your physical self and your behavior, will be born a new you. Let your mind be filled with a new positivism, a new strength, and a revitalized optimism. (6) Once you have delineated honest, valid outcomes, concentrate on them with all your might. What could be as easy and natural as drinking water? But stay focused lest you stray. (7) See the world as full of possibilities, full of marvelous changes. All you need to do is act on your authentic impulses, once you have determined them, and set sail for the sunrise. (8) Your right intentions should be on reinvigorating your body and spirit. Avoid the pitfalls of phantom hungers and illusory paths.

AVOID ILLUSIONS

False desires are self-defeating because they can never be satisfied. They always lead the individual to frustration. We can never come to possess that which is exterior to ourselves. Our desires attach themselves to the objects of our appetites: power, possessions, the perfect figure, the ideal relationship—and leave us desperate in our failure to obtain them. Erroneous appetites create desperation that is only relieved by our releasing the objects of our desires, then reorienting our attention to our true internal self. This mental discipline allows us to see things as they really are, not as they appear on TV and in magazine ads. This regaining of the self-control of our own minds leads to spiritual development, diminishing the impact of suffering, and deepening the virtues of compassion, moderation, and calm. Insight and wisdom are attained as one travels the route of morality, mental discipline and intuitive insight.

Be very careful what you yearn for. In this world of instant gratification, it is too easy to reach into the refrigerator or cupboard and pull out something that has the appearance of the object of our desires, but turns out to be pure illusion. It is as if we were on a perpetual merry-go-round, devouring peanuts, popcorn, and cotton candy in the carnival of life. Yet our hunger is never satisfied; moreover, our general health wanes and declines. You might just as well fertilize your garden with pretzels and root beer—it might just get by, but will never thrive and reach its potential. Those other noble goals of a reduced waistline, heightened senses, and the effortless will to achieve—go by the wayside. Without the proper beginnings, the voyage is aborted, hopes shattered, reality becomes a black hole where all our effervescent joy and optimism disappear.

Water is a mantra, a life force. It is ambrosial, the fluid that dissolves away the illusions of foodstuffs impersonating true nutriments. Once we truly believe in its key role in our lives, we become awakened. Our suffering diminishes, a calm spreads from our inner self out through the body to the outer world. We come to grips with ourselves as we achieve peace with the cosmos.

Karma (i.e., deed or act) is both the act that is performed as well as the results of that act. Siddhartha declared that a good act produces good fruit from that action, while bad fruit results from bad action. For there to be karma, there must be intention, which is even more important than the act itself. In fact, intention by itself produces karma, even when there is no acting out of that intention.

By acting out our H2O Diet, an energy surges through us. The interplay of our targeted intentions and the realization of those intentions becomes an organic whole: karma. We create our own metamorphosis, becoming the fruit of our own actions.

LIFE IS FLUX

All of reality is in constant change, all elements continually becoming something else. This vibrant shifting and re-arranging of the parts is in contrast to our sense of permanence, of things being eternally fixed. The stability that is so apparent to the senses is an illusion. Only by our denying the permanence of things do we achieve the destruction of selfish desires and egoism. Everything that inhabits our world is the sum of its parts, its aggregates. The Five Aggregates are: (1) the material body, composed of earth, fire, water and wind, as well as their by-products; the mental energies of: (2) sensation caused by contact through the senses—eyes, ears, nose, tongue, body and mind; (3) perception, realized through the notions of colors, sounds, odors, tastes, tangible things, and objects of thought; (4) the predisposition concerning colors, sounds, odors, tastes, tangible things, and objects of thought; (5) consciousness experienced as knowledge ascertained by the eyes, ears, nose, tongue, body and mind.

Because the underlying principle of life is change, we are dealt the ideal medium to become who we wish. We only lack imagination...and will. No radical changes are necessary to begin the process of life style changes—nothing threatening nor difficult nor complicated is involved. Our selfish desires and self-indulgences are impediments to be confronted comfortably and rationally. Never reproach or deride yourself. Each of us is a world of potential perfection, merely waiting to be realized. Be good to yourself, and that goodness will radiate from you.

Humans are an infinitely complex array of aggregates: (1) the material body is constructed from the earth elements, the spirit that burns within us, the air we breathe, and the water that courses through our veins; (2) the consciousness of ourselves reflected in our perceptions of what lies without, interpreted by our senses—simply return to your senses; trust them to reveal forgotten tastes and subtleties; (3) open your senses as if you were just awakening into this reality; revel in the explosive sweetness of a fresh orange, the inviting texture of a ripe strawberry, the luxuriant shades of forest green lettuce, the rich smell of fresh-fried chicken, the mystical transparency of a swirling glass of water; (4) flee the predisposition to colors, sounds, tastes, odors, ideas—take a fresh breath of life, opening your eyes to the wonders that float about you, as if you were a new-born engaged in the miracles unfolding at your fingertips; (5) your new consciousness will invite you to unfold as a lotus greeting the sun with open arms. At first, water will be startlingly alluring, and then so will be fruits, vegetables, and the endless array of nature's cornucopia that lays invitingly before you.

FREEDOM

Siddhartha pictured our flowing life stream as a river whose coarse is defined by its banks, yet whose water is constantly in flux. Its course is set by society and the nature of the reality that surrounds us, yet there is a constant rearranging of its internal structure, a constant evolving and flowing onward. Our personal nature is similar to that of a flame that, while transferred from one candle to another, remains constant while ever changing. Our desires are like that flame, ever burning, fueled by the objects around us. Yet once we confess to ourselves that we can never possess the objects of those desires, and indeed, once we come to realize that our pursuit of them is a false path leading only to frustration and misery, the false flame that burns our souls simply flickers out for lack of fuel. He called the cessation of these desires "nirvana," the state where all human cravings and desires are extinguished. Once we reach nirvana, our souls awaken.

Although we are swept along the stream of life, we are free to swim about. It is that freedom that allows us to choose an alternate reality, to improve our lot in life. But first we must elect with our own free will to remove ourselves from the quagmire of habit and custom. To do that, we do not have to swim against the current, nor force ourselves much to deviate from our course. It is not predestined that we should be chained to an arid diet of poisonous spirits and ruinous rubbish in plastic bags. Freedom begins by recognizing the futility of clinging to past injurious habits, and by actively seeking the enlightenment of water and a sound diet. Nirvana—where all absurd, irrelevant human cravings and desires are extinguished—awaits us just downstream.

48

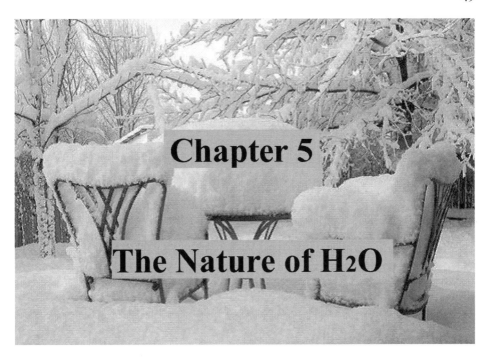

Chapter 5

The Nature of H₂O

IN THE BEGINNING

To the best of our understanding, the universe is in a perpetual cycle of birth, expansion, contraction, death, then back to the beginning for rebirth, and the continued repetition ad infinitum. Our current moment is some 14 billion years after the big bang, far from the projected end/beginning when gravity hurls the whole of the 100 billion galaxies into oblivion some 75 billion years after it all begins with the original implosion/explosion. Our own tiny planet is a speck of iron and assorted elements, a member of a family of fellow planets orbiting a medium-sized star, itself a member of the Milky Way Galaxy, a whirlpool of some 200 billion stars. It is indeed difficult for the senses to grasp the size and time framework of the next dimension, to envision the immense distances measured in millions and billions of light years.

After the initial fury of the primordial explosion of the universe, atoms began to congeal out of the electric plasma, but not for hundreds of thousands of years. These simple units of material, composed of a heavy proton orbited at a relatively huge distance by its electron, are the simplest of all atoms, hydrogen. Clouds of these atoms trillions of miles in extension congealed to give birth to stars. After billions of years of intense combustion, once a star burns out of its hydrogen-helium fuel and can no longer resist its own gravity, it collapses inwards, then explodes, spewing out its outermost layers to form most of the elements. Clouds of dust and fine particles eventually go into orbit around other stars. Gravity tugs relentlessly at them, pulling them together, condensing them into proto-planets—ones with iron cores near the adopted sun, and gaseous masses further out.

As vast amounts of electrical energy (i.e., lightning and volcanoes) energized the surface of our infant molten planet, hydrogen atoms were forced into a fixed relationship with oxygen, an atom composed of 16 heavy bodies at its core (8 protons and 8 neutrons), orbited by 8 electrons (i.e., particles of electricity at the distance and size a group of bumblebees would be from home plate if they were buzzing around the center field fence in a baseball park). When two sets of hydrogen twins are forced into a union with one set of oxygen twins, two water molecules are born: $2H_2 + O_2 = 2H_2O$. This tiny family, the H_2O molecule, is the cornerstone of life on earth.

A water molecule is just over 1 ten millionth of a millimeter across (1 mm. is about 1 twenty-fifth of an inch). Ten million water molecules stretched out end-to-end, would barely measure 1 millimeter. The two hydrogen atoms are separated by only 106 degrees, resulting in a positive charge on their end of the water molecule, and a negative charge on the oxygen's end of the molecule. In the frozen state, the molecules line up just like magnets—negative charge aligned with positive charge. As they heat up, these bonds are overcome by the kinetic energy of the vibrating molecules, and float about freely as water. Once reaching the temperature of 212 degrees Fahrenheit (100 degrees Celsius), water need only receive 540 calories of energy per gram to break completely free of its neighbors.

As it breaks its chains, the water molecule explodes up into the air as water vapor. If you should be unfortunate enough to come into contact with it in its vaporous state, it would condense, depositing its 540 calories per gram on your skin, giving you a nasty burn. Conversely, when you sweat, the evaporating water carries away 540 calories per gram as it evaporates. Our refrigerators work on the same principle: expanding gas on the closed interior of the refrigerator steals heat from the air, which is then led away to where a fan outside the refrigerator blows the heat away, as a pump compresses the gas for a return trip.

Contained gases normally maintain a distance of 10 times their diameter between themselves. Yet, when free to roam about, they tend to ride upwards on heat waves of air pushed out of the way by cooler air, which occupies less volume. Steam rises to become clouds that rain and snow. And just how many molecules of H_2O are there in a raindrop or a snowflake?

PROPERTIES

Once a gravitational-electrical stability is reached in this family of atoms, the new molecule assumes its own peculiar shape and properties. At temperatures at or below 32 degrees Fahrenheit (0 degrees Celsius), the molecules become stuck to one another, and the volume of the mass becomes increased by 15%. Water must lose 80 calories per gram to convert from its liquid state to a solid one, resulting in a solid as tough as rock.

52

In this crystalline state, the hydrogen bonds take precedence over all the other intermolecular forces. Those ice cubes you put in your drink must absorb 80 calories for every gram of their weight (there are 28 grams in an ounce) to break those bonds and convert themselves back into water.

The molecules in water in the liquid state cling to one another with the same hydrogen bonds as exist in its solid state, yet the energy they absorbed converting from ice to water allows them to keep active enough to maintain most of the bonds at bay. Water reaches its minimum volume at 39 degrees Fahrenheit (4 degrees Celsius), and then begins to expand as it heats up. Because of the ions (i.e., charged particles produced by the decomposition of water into H+ and OH-) floating around in it, water conducts electricity over a million times more than most other nonmetallic liquids at room temperature.

Water is a key element in the body's electrochemical processes, including not only nerve impulses, but also embracing higher reasoning. It is an efficient solvent for a variety of substances, but especially for those that disassociate to form ions. It is capable of purifying those substances, and of carrying out reactions involving them. If water is essential in allowing soaps to dissolve greases and filth from dirty dishes and clothes, it seems logical that water carries out similar functions within our own bodies. Water can enhance the oxidizing properties of other oxidizing agents. Lying on the surface of iron, water allows oxygen to unite with iron, forming rust (FeO_2). The red blood cells in our blood stream contain iron, which "rusts" when it comes into contact with the air we breathe into our lungs. This oxygen is carried to the cells to oxidize (i.e., burn) bits of food, releasing the energy essential to bodily functions. In exchange, carbon dioxide (CO_2) is returned from the cells to the lungs to be exhaled.

Hydrolysis is the decomposition or alteration of a chemical substance by water. Substances with strong acid or base characteristics tend to react with water. Probably the most common use of hydrolysis technology is in the production of soap. It begins with a fat, glyceryl stearate acid, being hydrolyzed with water to yield stearic acid and glycerin. Next, the stearic acid is neutralized with caustic soda to yield sodium stearate (i.e., soap) and water.

Starches, the reserve carbohydrates of plants, are usually stored in their seeds, roots or stems. Hydrolysis allows our bodies to convert these starches to sugars, which in turn supply energy to be stored, or used in muscular, digestive, and mental activities.

THE WATER AROUND US

Just as water is an internal constituent essential for our bodily functions, it is also the major component of our earth's processes. Most of the earth's crust is covered by water in its liquid and solid forms, as well as the water vapor that saturates the air we breathe and paints the skies white with clouds. The sun heats the oceans and the landmasses, daily evaporating millions of tons of steam into the atmosphere. The irregular heating of the earth's surface drives the more voluminous hot air nearer the equator to mix with the less voluminous cold air nearer the poles. By a complex process of solar heating, gravity and the earth's rotation on its axis, weather is created—a ceaseless exchange and distribution of water in the form of snow, ice, rain, currents, and vapor.

Water is virtually everywhere under, on, and above the surface of the earth. There are 1,400,000,000 cubic kilometers of it on Earth, 70% of which is locked into the form of ice. It is a necessary component of all life forms. In terms of human society, it is essential for all urban, agricultural, and industrial development. Unfortunately, water is a gregarious, at times a turbulent entity that invites pollution, complicating its use. It nourishes plants and animals, yet in hurricanes and tornadoes, as well as heavy rains, snows, and hailstorms, it can cause severe damage and loss of life. Rivers flood, dams burst, homes and populations are inundated and washed away. Businesses, homes, and cars as well as crops can be ruined, soils made infertile, and even sediments can disrupt streams, lakes, and harbors.

Mankind is in a constant struggle with nature to control unwanted flooding, erosion, pollution, water-borne diseases, and contamination. The stability of our economic existence, not to mention the health of ourselves and our planet, depends on coming to terms with nature's vicissitudes, understanding the dynamic ebb and flow of weather, the forces unleashed upon us, and the blessings she brings.

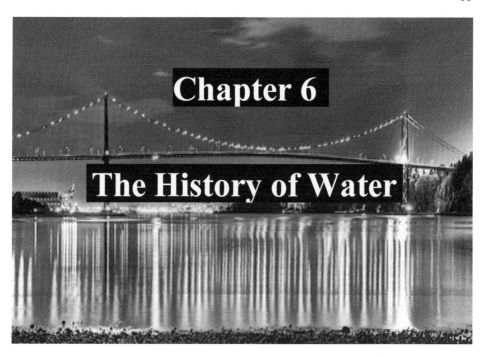

Chapter 6

The History of Water

TIME MACHINE

Imagine taking a trip in a time machine that transported you back through time to the Neolithic period (i.e., the New Stone Age) of our history. Your tribe would be an extended family, living out in the elements, with very fundamental needs: clothing, food, shelter, and water. You would naturally seek out the sources to satisfy those needs, devising implements to help you capture and butcher animals for food and skins; gather roots and berries; use trees, bushes, animal skins, and stones to build shelters; and exploit a convenient water source nearby. Fish and other inhabitants of water would be a welcome addition to your diet. Clay could be molded into vessels to transport and store water. A cool bath would be refreshing. Irrigation would allow your tribe to grow crops and assure its survival. All waste products could be washed away in a nearby river. Canoes could be fashioned from bark, bushes, and animal pelts, allowing you easy transportation to explore and exploit your environment, as well as trade with neighboring tribes who were also found living alongside a convenient water source. Even a watering hole would bring you in contact with a limitless supply of game.

Our earliest record of civilizations finds them located on the fringes where water meets land. Mesopotamia, for example, lies in the valley between the Tigris and the Euphrates rivers in modern-day Iraq. The development of agriculture made possible a sophisticated social organization that spawned a written language to codify everything from trade agreements and laws to religious dogma. This political, economic, religious, and military order allowed early man to extend his power and influence far beyond his cities. Resources were tracked, recorded, and controlled. The resulting accumulation of wealth was reflected in the architecture, clothing, and food of the inhabitants. Huge armies controlled an extended area, and religious, social, literary, and artistic influences spread outward from this epicenter.

Sumer, a region in the lower valley of the Euphrates river, emerged as a series of walled-in city-states beginning around 3000 B.C. Their magnificent palaces and multitiered temples were imitated as far away as the Mediterranean. The city-states were finally unified about 2320 B.C. by Saragon the Great from Akkad, who, once done conquering Sumer, washed his weapons in the waters of the Arabian Gulf to symbolize the end of warfare. Water is a marvelous cleansing agent, as well as a ready symbol for atonement, purity, sanctity, and change—even life itself.

Other cultures soon emerged along rivers, streams, lakes, and oceans: the Indus Valley civilization of India around 2700 B.C.; the Minoans of Crete, around 2200 B.C.; the Shang civilization in China, around 1766 B.C.; and the Olmecs in Mexico, around 1200 B.C.

EGYPT

Like Mesopotamia and the Indus, the North African civilization that arose along Egypt's Nile River prior to 3000 B.C. owed its existence to their watery lifeline that cut a green swath through the desert. The Blue Nile, which originates in Ethiopia, meets the White Nile from Uganda in Khartoum, then flows northward for 1900 miles to empty into the Mediterranean. Those who lived by its banks prospered, and were protected by the endless desert that surrounds the narrow green band of the Nile that extends from 1 mile, up to 13 miles from its shores. As this mystical river flows into Egypt at Aswan, it falls into the first of its six cataracts. In the last 100 miles of its journey, it fans out into the marshy flatlands of the delta. Once a year, the Nile gushed over its banks, pregnant with the torrential rains of Ethiopia. Towns became islands, yet at the same time, thousands of tons of fertile silt were being deposited on their land. A vital source of irrigation was a stone's throw away.

After the floods, a simple application of geometry reasserted the individual's property lines. In years of drought, famine followed. The first calendar was a reflection of the life-giving seasons: "Inundation," "Emergence of the fields from the water," and "Drought." As the population grew and became more cohesive, more social planning evolved. The division of labor beat to the pulse of the river. During the Emergence, men were employed to trap and store the abundant water. They turned their attention to harvesting and threshing during the Drought. And during the Inundation, they were freed to labor on quarrying, transporting, and erecting the massive stones for the pharaoh's magnificent pyramids and holy centers.

The Nile was Egypt's wealth. The nation's power was determined by its agricultural success. As such, water had to be carefully nurtured. Dikes were constructed to protect population centers. Huge catch basins were excavated to trap the receding floodwaters. Intricate canals branched out from these basins to the fields. Wells were sunk to further provide for the needs of the populace. The land that was annually flooded became valuable real estate. Courts were busy determining water rights. Even in the afterlife, the dead were asked if they had been guilty of detaining water from its rightful course. Wheat flowed out of this fertile, administered land. All along the Nile, but especially in the Delta swamps, papyrus thrived. From ancient times to the 12th Century A.D., Egyptians practiced a lucrative monopoly by producing paper from this grass-like plant by soaking, pressing, and drying thin slices of its pith. The remaining fibers of papyrus were fashioned into rope, baskets, mats, sandals, and a hundred other products.

With this abundance of water and food, Egyptian farmers found it a relatively simple task to raise cattle, pigs, and goats. In the Delta, reed boats were used in the trapping of geese, ducks, and cranes. Quantities of fish were captured with nets. The Nile Valley produced an abundance of castor oil, flaxseed oil, and sesame oil. This oil was essential not only for cooking, but also for burning in lamps, and even for cleaning oneself. Even the mud could be dried in the sun, and used to create everything from walls and ovens to humble homes and palaces. These all in turn became products easily distributed by water. Bricks, pigs, oils, and wheat could be piled on papyrus boats that reached the length of the Nile, and far beyond to the Roman, Greek and Phoenician shores of the Mediterranean.

GREECE

Across some 600 miles of the Mediterranean, northwest from the Nile Delta, lies the fractured empire of Greece. Due to favorable sailing conditions, Greeks early on learned to follow the winds to the neighboring islands that dot the Aegean Sea between Greece and modern Turkey. Beginning around 1100 B.C., the Greek city-states began to establish colonies, first along the coasts and nearby islands, then all the way from Spain, Gaul, and Italy, up into the Black Sea, and down to the North African coast. Trade and expansion were made possible by the sea, and by harbors and rivers that afforded easy inland access. The colonies all spoke the same language, and shared in common epic songs and stories that had been inherited from antiquity. These stories, related by bards such as Homer, were not only entertaining, but also inspirational history, picturing their ancestors as strong, brave, and noble. The cast of characters included mythical gods and heroes, and amazing deeds and adventures.

Poseidon (Neptune to the Romans), the god of the sea, was one of the most widely worshiped of the Greek gods. Homer ascribed to him his aqueous realm, as well as he had ascribed those realms of Zeus—the sky, and Hades, the underworld. They all shared Mt. Olympus and the earth. Depending on his whim, Poseidon calmed the seas or created tempests. Sailors and fishermen prayed to him, and many coastal settlements were given his name. Inland, his cult inhabited clefts in rocks, pools, streams, and springs. The farmers' success with his crops depended on maintaining his good graces. His sculpted figure—that of a stern, mature male, is found on the west pediment of the Parthenon, contending with Athena. With the Gorgon Medusa, he begot Pegasus, the winged horse, who was associated with the springs of the ocean. Stallions, bulls, and sheep were sacrificed to him. Poseidon means literally, "Husband of the Earth."

ROME

Just west of Greece, Italy juts down into the Mediterranean like a woman's boot, its toe nearly touching Sicily, itself a mere 100 miles across open waters to Carthage, the Phoenician colony in Northern Africa. Roman culture originally was Etruscan, a loose agglomeration of city-states clustered in the Po River valley in the north of Italy, which flourished as early as the 6th century B.C. The Etruscans were seafaring traders, plying the Mediterranean principally to Phoenicia and Greece. From them, the Romans learned the art of hydraulic engineering, eventually constructing mammoth stone aqueducts throughout the Roman Empire. Resulting from water-borne trade, the alphabet borrowed from Phoenicia and Greece spawned literacy, literature, a body of laws, and the sciences.

From its humble beginnings as a city-state on the Tiber River in the 3rd century B.C., by the 3rd century A.D., Roman influence had spread throughout the Mediterranean basin, north to Gaul and Scotland, and into the Near East. Technological advances, such as concrete, allowed massive buildings and complexes. As cities grew, and the population exploded, ships were mobilized to transport goods and foodstuffs, especially grains, to Rome from throughout its empire.

At the heart of each of the Roman cities was a sophisticated drainage system, as well as the omnipresent aqueducts. Water distribution was in private hands and, although satisfactory, never approached modern standards. With no efficient valves or pumps, leakage was around 50 percent. The hallmark of Roman sophistication, the civic fountain, was in fact an outlet for the temporary overflow of water. Public baths were constructed at public expense on a grand scale designed to please the emperor's tastes, but also by commercial private enterprises for public use. These baths served as social gathering places, as well as pure entertainment. Ornate complexes of hot and cold rooms were made possible by the technological advancements of waterproof plaster, glazed tiles, and central heating beneath the floors.

MEXICO

In Mexico, high in a southern central valley, where once lay a glittering silver lake, now lies Mexico City, a mega-metropolis of some 20 million souls. Around 1325, a desperate Chichimec tribe wandered into the verdant valley, searching for a haven from the barren semi-desert conditions of their homeland. These people we call Aztecs (they called themselves Mexica), forced themselves onto a swampy island in the shallow Lake Texcoco. Their prophecy had described their destination as one where they would find an eagle perched on a cactus, devouring a snake. There they were soon to extend their island by building a series of small floating islands of floating reeds and water lilies covered with silt from the lake's bottom, with interconnecting canals. These served as gardens that produced corn, squash, beans, chili, and an array of vegetables and flowers. Later they would raise massive stone pyramids, atop which they would nourish the sun with sacrificial victims.

This miserable band at first survived by fishing, and searching the tall reeds for eggs, snakes, and other vermin. By the time Hernán Cortés arrived with his conquistadors in 1519, the Aztec's capital of Tenochitlán had grown to a population of 200,000 that controlled most of central Mexico. They wrote their history in deerskin books, codified laws, stimulated arts and crafts, music, and poetry, trading as far away as the Pacific and Caribbean coasts, Central America, and north to Texas, where they maintained a system of tribute by military might. A long dike was erected across Lake Texcoco to keep the turbid water from their floating gardens, which were fed by Lake Chalco. A stone aqueduct was constructed from Chapultepec to the island city of Tenochtitlán. In the city center they built a series of brightly painted temples and palaces, the most elaborate being the twin pyramid dedicated to the bloody war god, Huitzilopochtli, and the rain god, Tláloc.

A society that fails in agriculture suffers from famine, and eventually disappears. Water is the liquid that makes civilization flow. Their god of rain and the heavens, Tláloc, literally symbolized "he who makes things grow." Besides representing water, he was associated with snakes, mountains, flooding, drought, hail, ice, and lightning. His carved image covers pyramids and ceremonial centers, and can be readily recognized by the rings around his eyes, snake fangs jutting down from his mouth, and his butterfly moustache.

When the earth begins to warm in the spring, snakes arouse from their winter-cave hibernations, and seek the open air. Thus snakes came to symbolize the rebirth of the earth, coming as they did from its bowels. Being a god with snake-like fangs, Tláloc was not a god to be easily reckoned with. His ringed eyes signified the renewal of vegetation in the spring, achieved by sacrificing a human victim.

To an agricultural people so entwined with the rhythms of nature, Tláloc's heaven is depicted as a sanctuary with bountiful rains, tropical flowers, and butterflies fluttering about. It is pictured in wall paintings with a gyrating mob of human figures prancing about, jesting in word glyphs, and swimming in abundant waters. Tláloc, as the reigning deity of this paradise, stoically wears his butterfly moustache as a promise of things to come. In 1964, when the 168-ton stone monolith of Tláloc was moved to Chapultepec Park near the entrance to the National Museum of Anthropology, a deluge of rain fell in torrents unprecedented in the history of Mexico City.

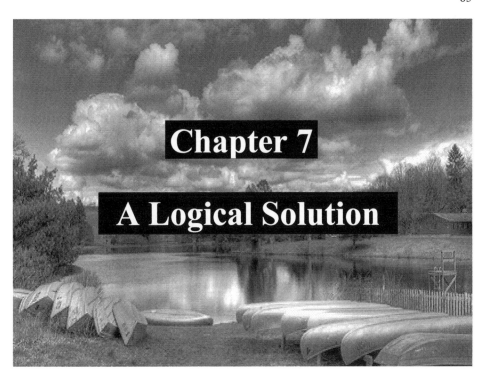

Chapter 7

A Logical Solution

WHAT PRICE SUCCESS?

Joyce is a young professional with a husband and two children. She was raised with common-sense values, and an inbred determination to make her mark on the world. She did so at first by a perseverant application of her energies to her high school curriculum, then by doggedly pursuing a college degree. Her parents were not able to pay completely for her university studies, so she had to supplement the tuition, board and room costs with a part-time job, and eventually a series of small scholarships. Her diet was erratic at best during this monastic period of her life, and she chronically suffered from hypertension. She skipped meals, ate on the run, and gulped down junk food at every turn.

As Joyce determinedly enhanced her mind, and moved toward fulfillment of her dream of a professional degree, she ignored the very source of her success—her body and, ultimately, her mind. If you set about breeding a thoroughbred horse for competitive racing, logic tells you to give him a diet high in nutrition, low in fats (not to mention sugars), provide him with plenty of water, exercise him regularly, and rest him when indicated. What is so transparent for an animal's care, is so easily overlooked when we care for ourselves. Are we truly making the right choices for the desired outcome?

COFFEE VS. WATER

These may sound like hollow words of advice to a blooming intellectual on her way to establishing her niche in the world, but Joyce ignored an essential ingredient in her recipe for success: water. She was up early in the morning to attack her day with vigor. A cup of strong coffee stimulated her mind, but destroyed her stomach, and actually dehydrated her, depriving her body of its natural cleansing and operating agent. It seemed she was on a treadmill, never being able to keep pace with the demands she placed upon herself, nor catch up on the sleep she so efficiently denied herself. No wonder she was so worn out both physically and mentally.

If she would have stopped and thought about the nature of her bodily functions, and been more considerate of her needs, Joyce would have begun her day with a light breakfast, topped off with a glass of water. At vital intervals throughout her hectic day, a glass of water here and there would have revitalized her and kept her energies operating at an optimal level. She chose, instead, to gulp down quantities of coffee and caffeinated soft drinks to stimulate her performance.

Little did Joyce consider the nature of caffeine: it is a drug, a bitter, crystalline alkaloid that prolongs the stimulating effects of cyclic AMP (adenosine monophosphate) in the heart and central nervous system. (AMP is a crystalline nucleotide vital to the energy processes of all living cells; it is also a major regulator of the cell's biochemical activity.) She should have listened to Mark, one of her high school friends, who had experimented with a potpourri of drugs: for all the pleasure and heightened energy drugs give you at the moment, they sooner or later demand back payment in full, plus interest. Every artificially wakeful moment, every ounce of productivity gained, your system will take back by reduced awareness, disorientation, and even a total shutdown.

Caffeine is a drug not to be taken lightly, and even in low doses, it is often a desirable mild stimulant. If Joyce would have drunk her wakeup cup of coffee, then soon followed it with a piece of fruit and a glass of water, her body could have detoxified itself naturally, and she could have regained an equilibrium that would carry her on through her day at an optimal level. Think, Joyce, think!

Joyce was so busy with academics and trying to shuffle the needs of her personal life with her own expectations and the demands placed on her, that she denied herself a key element of her success: water. It sounds almost trivial, somehow unimportant, but if you are in the process of building a great edifice, it is not wise to place fragile bricks right at your foundation. It is amazing how clever and astute we can be, yet how totally unaware of what constitutes the healthy you. What element do you suppose is a component of every vital process that occurs in the human body—coffee?

When we lie down at night for our 8-hour fast, does the body completely shut down? Obviously not. We carry on metabolic processes that reduce our nutrients—the carbohydrates, proteins, and fats we ingest during the day, to smaller, absorbable units like sugars, amino acids, and fatty acids. The digestive enzymes and acids from the salivary glands, pancreas, and liver are awash in our digestive tract in a river of H_2O. The heart continues incessantly pumping blood throughout our systems. The lungs breathe, inhaling the oxygen essential in breaking down our food, and exhaling the carbon dioxide that is the byproduct of that chemical process.

By paying sporadic attention to her physical needs, Joyce managed to consume sufficient quantities of vitamins and minerals, but undernourished herself by failing to consume sufficient water. H_2O. Not coffee, tea, soda, lemonade, orange juice, or one of dozens of fortified drinks. Accept no substitutes. The answer is transparently simple, but so much so, that it is easily overlooked.

How much effort would it have taken Joyce to remedy her dilemma? Very little. But awareness is the first step to success. We have all elevated our lives at key moments by an insightful awareness that basically changed the way we live. When you cut your finger, wash it, apply an antiseptic, then a band-aid, your chances of curing yourself are greatly enhanced. That is common sense, logical, and undeniable. Yet how many children and even adults fail to follow that procedure? And if you fail to implement that strategy, where does it inevitably lead? If you have an important exam or you are going to compete in an athletic event, it makes sense to go to bed early the night before.

It even makes sense to establish a habit of satisfying your body's elementary needs by getting into the habit of sufficient sleep. There are a thousand excuses for burning the candle at both ends, but few are legitimate. And, ultimately, you pay the piper. Fatigue leads to reduced performance, mental fogginess and lapses of memory. When you train yourself for that big race, think of your racehorse and his needs: sound food, sufficient exercise, rest, and adequate water. It just makes sense to optimize your performance by establishing a routine based on practical logic.

FAT

Besides chronic fatigue, Joyce suffered from an accumulation of baby fat. She ascribed it to her sedentary lifestyle, which was a valid assumption, but rationalized that there were too few hours in her day to rectify her condition. She was wrong. All she needed to have done is spend a few moments analyzing her lifestyle objectively, make a reasonable plan, and act on it. Joyce could have considered a short walk once or twice a day, not only to reinvigorate the body, but also to clear out some of the cobwebs in her mind, permitting sounder concentration and a higher degree of awareness.

She could have optimized her exercise by consuming a glass of water before that walk, and another glass upon arriving back home. Few people would dream of trapping their pets in a cage or at a desk for 8 hours a day without allowing them a walk to stimulate their bodily functions, not to mention their spiritual well-being. Not only would Joyce have felt better about herself, seeing her clothes fit a little nicer and herself reflected wholesome in her mirror, but she also would have simplified her academic and social performances.

There are usually logical reasons people feel bloated, constipated, muddled, and feeble. One reason may be immobility, brought on by a real lack of desire and motivation. But is it not also plausible that a dehydrated body has a reduced spirit, virtually unable to cure itself? It is almost revolutionary to consider that the quality of your life can be redeemed by a glass of water. It is not *the* element in a winning diet, but an undeniably essential component. What we need often is just a plan—one born of our own imagination, shared with us by a friend or guru, or accessed from a source like TV, the Internet, or a book or magazine. But why do the purported answers have to be so convoluted and incomprehensible? The simple answer is the sure answer: drink sufficient water, and a chain effect will take place that will cleanse the body, overhaul the mental circuitry, and motivate the soul to action. Just try it.

STRESS

One of the most common ailments of our modern society is stress. Most stress-related diseases involve cardiovascular or gastrointestinal functions. The majority of people whose bodies suffer from these malfunctions are unaware that they are victims of an aberrant stress factor. For the cardiovascular system to meet the tissues' varying demands for oxygen, nutrients, and the elimination of metabolic wastes, it must constantly be altering its functioning. It is well-documented that threatening situations greatly increase the cardiac output, while only slightly increasing the oxygen consumption, throwing the body's equilibrium out of balance. Pain or fright can cause the heartbeat to accelerate anywhere from 10 beats per minute up to 50 beats per minute.

Because the kidneys perform the function of controlling blood pressure by the secretion of sodium, they too can be impaired by the altered cardiovascular state. When one feels threatened, sodium is retained in the blood plasma, resulting in an acute elevation of blood pressure and, over the long run, hypertension, and eventually even heart disease and stroke. Also, various hormones are released to prepare the body to deal with the stressful stimulus. One of these is epinephrine, released by the adrenal gland to stimulate the cardiovascular system and facilitate metabolism. Stress can readily push your body into a crisis, and eventually, serious damage can be done.

By the age of 60, approximately 20% of the population must cope with high blood pressure. It is undetermined how many of them actually suffer their abnormal blood-pressure levels from the inherited tendency (as opposed to a conditioned tendency) to overreact to stressful situations. Yet it is known that those whose heartbeat rises dramatically when confronted by a challenging situation, usually react to similar situations in the same way. Any environmental event can trigger the stress reaction—that reaction increasing as the demand for the body to change increases. It is the intensity of the demand for change that is the key factor, not the type of demand in itself.

As Sir Isaac Newton noted: "Every body continues in a state of rest, or of uniform motion in a right line, unless it is compelled to change that state by forces impressed upon it." The nature of life on this earth *is* change, but we all resist change to varying degrees, and that resistance can seriously wear on our very being. Stress creates high blood pressure, which can then cause strokes, as well as other detrimental reactions.

Joyce made her way through high school and college on determination and adrenalin. She was hyperactive, often running on half a tank. Her reserves were depleted, and she often found herself in a fog. Having pushed herself beyond her natural limits thus far, there was no turning back. She landed a demanding job with the accompanying pressures and expectations. She was a success in both monetary and status-based terms, but seemed to be out of touch with herself.

After such prolonged stress on her body and mind, Joyce was setting herself up for a crash. Her intermittent vacations were exercises in futility. She was so wired she could never really enjoy the rest and calm that seemed to surround her, yet lay just out of her reach. And before she could get in touch with herself, she was back into the old grind. Weekends were work-and-worry times also, punctuated with survival errands, and catnaps on the sofa. She dragged herself through two years of this routine, depriving her body and soul of their basic nutrients. When her body cried out for a glass of water, she drowned herself in coffee, which dehydrated her body, and prolonged the vicious cycle. She was on a merry-go-round, but failed to imagine how to step off with grace. She was beginning to teeter on the edge of a black depression, not able to cope with the stress she herself had invited into her life.

Things seemed to change course when she accepted the marriage proposal of her college sweetheart, and soon found herself married and pregnant. The pregnancy was a hiatus from her colorless job, its incessant demands, as well as her own obstinate demands on herself. The artificial world she had found increasingly difficult to cope with, had suddenly been transformed into one of sense and promise. She tuned into her body's demands, and tried to satisfy them.

Her diet became sensible, and she followed her doctor's suggestion of rest, light exercise, a well-rounded diet, including carbohydrates, proteins, and fats, with plentiful amounts of fruits and vegetables—and 8 glasses of water a day. She initially substituted fruit juices and sodas for those nebulous 8 glasses of water, but slowly felt herself turn the corner to good health and sanity. Then came the birth of her baby, and soon upon his heels, postpartum depression.

When we suffer from stress, the hypothalamus secretes corticotropin-releasing hormone (CRH), which itself causes the release of hormones that rush cortisol into the bloodstream. Cortisol is a hormone that raises the sugar levels in the blood, helping the cardiovascular system retain a normal blood pressure. In the last trimester of pregnancy, the mother's placenta releases CRH into her bloodstream, tripling her blood-sugar levels. Once the baby is born and the placenta removed, the CRH levels in the bloodstream diminish dramatically, producing the clinical signs of depression. Only after a period of time does the hypothalamus return to its normal output of CRH.

Understanding this natural process, the average woman can deal with her postpartum depression by pursuing a normal diet of foods that provide her with: sufficient iron; calcium; thiamin; the antioxidant vitamins A, C, and E; niacin; riboflavin; and folic acid. She should be careful to avoid caffeine, alcohol, and excessive salt if at all possible. Responding to her urges to overeat, or consume sodas, coffee, or alcoholic drinks by instead drinking a glass of water, she can be assured she is on the right path to recovering her physical and mental equilibrium.

DEPRESSION

Depression springs from a multitude of sources: from radical changes in our life style, the loss of loved ones, hormone changes, illnesses, and chemical abuse, to erratic diets. It is difficult to cure ourselves when our defenses are severely depleted. Obviously, what we put into our bodies can severely aggravate our reaction to those problems that lead us away from a balanced state. The American Psychiatric Association assigns the following symptoms to depression: a poor, or increased appetite; insomnia; delayed movements or thoughts; fatigue; self-reproach and guilt; lack of decision and concentration; and thoughts of death and suicide.

At one time or another, all of us are subject to this negative energy state, which ranges from sadness to a deep depression. In fact, about 15 percent of the population occasionally slips into the deep mire of distress. To keep ourselves on an even keel while we attempt to maneuver through these difficult periods, we should attempt to focus on the light at the end of the tunnel, and move towards it a step at a time, a positive thought at a time. Try: A simple, well-rounded diet. A pleasant walk. A refreshing glass of water. Fortunately, Joyce learned of the importance of these options, and put them to the test. Once she became enlightened, she realized that all these elements contribute their share by keeping us from sinking into the abyss, by allowing us to heal from within. She was well on her way to recovery.

"Water is best."—Pindar

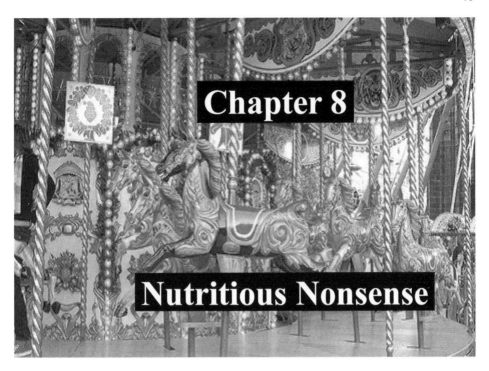

Chapter 8

Nutritious Nonsense

THE MEDICINE MAN

The medicine man rolled into town with his covered wagon painted brightly with promises of miraculous cures for all that ailed you—all attributed to a magic elixir he sold with a mysterious hype. His horses, having witnessed his performance a thousand weary times, waited patiently as he set up his show and began to draw a small crowd thirsty for entertainment of any kind. His pitch was straight from vaudeville and *The Music Man*: this Professor Harold Hill threw the fear of fire and brimstone into the audience with his warnings of gout, fatigue, and impotence, promising their remission with a slug or two from his dollar bottle of white lightning. As he waxed and waned, promises spewed out—of stimulating desired hair growth, eliminating the wrath of the common hangover, calming the upset stomach, relieving the aches and pains of an overstressed body, increasing endurance, creating an aura of physical attraction to subvert the opposite gender, eliminating rashes and the pain of snake bites, stimulating the appetite—or in fact reducing the appetite if that were the desire…and so on.

There was no ailment under the sun safe from the healing properties of Dr. Hill's Miracle Potion. If there would have been a truth-in-labeling law in effect, you might have discovered that Dr. Hill was brewing a magical potion in a bathtub from a water solution colored with boiled tealeaf extract, saturated with alcohol, and flavored with sugar. That, indeed, sounds like a recipe capable of curing just about anything that ails you.

The amazing thing is that Dr. Hill left a legacy to be inherited and enhanced by his grandchildren, one that permeates the airwaves, and is plastered on nearly every page of print, across billboards, two-thirds of the mail we receive, and the Internet pages we consult. We are being bombarded with propaganda that is every bit as inviting and misleading as Dr. Hill's snake bite remedy. Yet the advertising continues, because it is fed by voluminous sales to a virtual multitude of gullible consumers who seem to enjoy being convinced of the mystical properties, and taken in by the clever subconscious associations created in the advertising boardrooms. Everyone delights in the fantasy of the ultimate feather that delivers the ultimate tickle.

In our hysteria to reinvent ourselves in the image of stick-thin models, esthetically emaciated couples cavorting about on beaches and tanning salons with power drinks raised in toasts to the good life, and macho cowboys painting their lungs with brownish tars and nicotine, we get distracted from our real goal. These illusory vehicles all lead nowhere. They are mirages of advertising fantasies conjured up to sell products, not to enliven our existence on earth. Their secondary effects can be terribly distracting, if not downright devastating. We have to develop a critical, honest eye to evaluate the stream of chaotic information flowing through our senses, and discard the inessential, superfluous flotsam and jetsam. Let your true nature develop filtering criteria. Set your sights on real goals: Happiness. Health. Security. Love. Comfort.

SODA SUCCESS

Let's start by seriously thinking about the liquids we ingest by the gallon. Last year the average American drank 50 gallons of soda. Of course, you rationalize, that means only about a gallon a week. Those bottles and cans are everywhere. They occupy an entire aisle in every respectful supermarket on the planet. What is this pause that refreshes so heartily it has spread its web around the world, capturing the imagination of the world's population, and drowning us in a sea of effervescent pleasure? Could we be dealing here with nothing more at heart than flavored water with bubbles and a shot of caffeine? Probably. Yet that product, simple in concept as it may be, is the subject of an advertising blitz that would make Freud shudder.

Sodas have become icons of the material society anxious to find meaning in the mundane, and at the same time, represent immense profits in an ambrosial product. These magnificent bottles and cans are poised proudly on tables in Paris, Madrid, New York, Istanbul, Nairobi, Peking, and Moscow, lending an aura of exhilaration, invigoration, stimulation, and above all, refreshment to all fortunate enough to savor them. Pretty arrogant for a sugar buzz of carbonated water, caramel color, phosphoric acid, a potpourri of flavors, and that omnipresent caffeine punch.

Now take a closer look at an outstanding example of soda success. By the end of the twentieth century, Coca-Cola had penetrated 195 countries, where its annual sales topped $15 billion dollars (that is: nearly $3 for every living human being on the planet). That exponential growth had its humble beginnings in Atlanta, Georgia, in 1886, when Dr. John Pemberton converted his popular nerve tonic, stimulant, and headache remedy, "Pemberton's French Wine Coca," to Coca-Cola, by simply replacing the wine with sugar. The city fathers had passed a prohibition law that year, and the good doctor's response was simply to eliminate the alcohol from his formula. Contrary to popular folklore, the principal ingredients of his soft drink were neither the coca leaf nor the kola nut (the kola nut was the source for the caffeine that aimed at treating headaches).

Dr. Pemberton was in fact a handsome man, a doctor by the age of nineteen, an entrepreneur who created an outstanding laboratory for chemical analysis and manufacturing in Atlanta, while additionally managing the distribution of his French Wine Cola to nearly all the drugstores in the city. It was with little added effort that his Coca-Cola brand began to catch on in Atlanta. His first-year sales totaled a humble 3,200 servings. Today, many households probably top that number by themselves. By 1895 Coca-Cola was being sold in every state and territory in the United States. The rest is history.

ADDITIVES

And what of the major constituent in every soft drink and fruit juice consumed? Water, that innocuous yet powerful chemical agent, is the invisible force that gives body to a multitude of additive expressions. Yet how often is water found in its pure state? Even the common drinking water that runs out of the tap probably contains a good amount of dissolved minerals, and chlorine, put there to eradicate any threatening bacteria that might otherwise make its way into our bodies. In over 50% of our drinking water, fluoride is added in miniscule amounts (about 1 part per million) to inhibit the acidogenic plaque bacteria coating our teeth. It inhibits the growth of Streptococcus mutans that inhabit dental plaque, and also inhibits bacterial enzymes, reducing the amount of acid produced by the catabolism of fermentable carbohydrates.

Fluoride also attracts other minerals (like calcium), which build up the tooth mass, creating a layer even more resistant to bacteria than the original enamel. In short, it prevents cavities. For health reasons, or simply to enhance taste, carbonation is occasionally added, or may occur naturally, as is the case with trace substances. Magnesium sulfate, potassium chloride, potassium bicarbonate, and salt are often listed as ingredients on bottled-water labels. It may appear in a thousand disguises, sold under an equal number of brand names, but water is water. In a category by itself, it is the king of liquids. Do not let anyone try to convince you otherwise.

Your sugar needs are best satisfied with fresh fruits, not flavored water. Once you begin to appreciate the colorful variety of fresh fruits offered at your local supermarket, and bring them home to decorate your table, the nature of your body and spirit begins to change before your eyes. Present them in an easily accessed fruit bowl; serve them sliced as a snack or dessert. There is virtually no limit to the amount of fruits and vegetables you can consume with benefit.

CARBOHYDRATES

A multitude of casual as well as serious dieters swear by

the currently popular low-carbohydrate diet. But just what is the nature of carbohydrates, and how do they affect our metabolism? One simple form of carbohydrate is sugar. The process of photosynthesis in plants produces sugars by creating large molecules by combining water (H_2O) with carbon (C). The sugar molecule occurs in the form of $C_{12}H_{22}O_{11}$, sucrose (glucose and fructose joined together—found in sugar cane and sugar beets), and in other disaccharides such as maltose, and lactose; and $C_6H_{12}O_6$, fructose (found in fruits and honey), and in other monosaccharides such as glucose, and galactose. Starch, $(C_6H_{10}O_5)n$, is a complex carbohydrate (i.e., a polysaccharide), that can be easily degraded into sugar. It is found in abundance in seeds and roots: potatoes, rice, corn, wheat, cassava, and many vegetable foods. Even as starchy foods (breads, tortillas, pastas, crackers, and so on) are being chewed, the acids in our saliva are breaking them down into sugars.

Raw starches are difficult to digest because the carbohydrates are contained within the thin walls of the cells. Yet when moist heat swells the starch, the cell walls burst, exposing them to hydrolysis by amylolytic enzymes that convert the starch into soluble substances. The plant wall consists of a matrix of dietary fiber components interlinked with a variety of fellow carbohydrates, proteins, fats, and inorganic compounds. Although we cannot digest this fiber, it is key for normal gastrointestinal function.

The three nutrients that supply calories to the body are: carbohydrates, fats, and proteins. Diets that suggest a severe reduction or even an elimination of carbohydrates overlook their function in maintaining the healthy activity of the sympathetic nervous system, as well as that of supplying the brain with a constant supply of glucose. Because carbohydrates cannot be stored, except for limited amounts found in the liver and muscle as glycogen, they must be ingested on a consistent basis. If there are not sufficient carbohydrate levels, the brain begins to draw on the body's fat stores—creating a potentially dangerous condition called ketosis.

As carbohydrates are consumed, insulin production is stimulated. Insulin is essential in regulating the entry of glucose into cells and storing body fat, yet at high levels, can damage arterial walls. The key to maintaining an optimal level of insulin is to have a fit body and a healthy weight. When carbohydrates are reduced, calorie intake is restricted to fats and proteins. Yet too much fat intake can damage artery walls and promote heart disease. Too much animal protein wears the kidneys out while removing the waste products of protein metabolism. Also, the body benefits from the protective factors contained in the carbohydrate-rich foods that provide protection against cancer, heart disease, and other chronic illnesses.

Low-carb, high-protein diets promise you that the fat will melt away, along with the unwanted inches that fill out your clothing where you least want to see bulges. The most effective of these simple plans recommend reducing your carbohydrate intake and diminishing your hunger pangs and cravings by eliminating refined sugar, white rice, white bread, and crackers, and replacing them with fiber-rich whole fruits and vegetables, brown rice, and whole-wheat bread.

During the first two-week period, men are told to expect to lose up to 8 pounds, and women 6. These diets include basically healthy foods such as lean meat, poultry, seafood, low-fat cheese, eggs, and a variety of vegetables. Gradually, other foods are added: cereal, skim milk, and whole fruits, until finally the diet is broadened to include: wheat, multi-grain bread, whole-wheat pasta, beans, lentils, peas, and brown rice.

By strictly following the regimen, after the first two weeks, you should expect to lose up to 2 pounds per week.

A common-sense approach includes limiting your consumption of products that contain ground wheat and corn (e.g., bread, pasta, tortillas, etc.). These foods take up to six hours to digest. Stick with fruits and vegetables, rice and potatoes, as well as baked beans. These latter foods take less time to digest, and are packed with necessary vitamins and minerals. They also contain the fiber our digestive systems need to function properly.

FATS

Other diets focus on reducing fat intake. Fat lends much of the desirable flavor to foods, and because it takes more time to digest, gives a sensation of fullness. It contains 9 calories per gram, whereas protein and carbohydrate each contain 4 calories per gram. These diets recommend that saturated fats found in meats, dairy products, and partially hydrogenated oils should be replaced by unsaturated fats. Care must be taken to then increase the amount of fruits, vegetables, fiber, and whole grains consumed. By following these simple guidelines, one lowers the risk of heart disease, reduces hypertension, and the risk of certain cancers.

Exercise continues to be highly recommended to accompany the reduced fat consumption. Not only is weight lost by reducing fat intake, but also the body is placed under less stress by the reduced energy demanded to metabolize the fat. A word of caution: do not replace the lost fat consumption with sugar intake. Americans currently consume some 150 pounds of sugar per year. The goal should be to diminish not only the saturated fat use, but also the sugar intake, replacing them with fruits, vegetables, and fiber. Healthy fats are essential in a   balanced diet. Beware of donuts, and all that fried junk food, but continue using olive, corn, and canola oils to reduce the risk of heart disease. Excess body fat usually tags along with an excess of fats and carbohydrates, and the couch-potato syndrome.

PROTEIN

Many new diets recommend a high amount of protein to accompany the low carbohydrate intake. All animals from protozoa to homo sapiens need to ingest protein in their diets. The word protein itself reveals its importance: it is from Greek, *protos*, meaning "first." Some lower life forms can synthesize their own carbon-skeleton proteins, and even we can synthesize some of its constituent amino acids from carbon and nitrogen precursors. But others must be culled from the food we eat as our digestive systems pulverize it, freeing up the protein molecules formed from a complex arrangement of amino acids. These amino acids contain carbon, hydrogen, oxygen, nitrogen, often sulfur, and occasionally phosphorus, iron, iodine, and other elements.

After digestion, the amino acids can become an integral part of our body's: protoplasm (a semi-liquid, viscous, translucent colloid—the essential living matter of all living cells), enzymes (organic catalysts for chemical reactions in the body), hemoglobin (the iron-based red coloring in red blood cells that carries oxygen to the cells from the lungs, then makes the return trip with carbon dioxide to be breathed out), bone, and skin. Some of the amino acids that are not removed from the bloodstream to be integrated into body tissue are quickly disassembled to satisfy the body's need for energy; others become fat; while still others are simply excreted. Our bodies are not capable of storing proteins, so we must ingest foods containing the eight essential amino acids daily.

Protein is found in abundance in red meat, chicken, fish, milk, eggs, legumes (i.e., peas and beans), and nuts. Because of the saturated fats and high cholesterol levels it contains, consumption of red meat should be kept to a minimum. Studies indicate it contributes to colon cancer and heart disease. If you are concerned about your calcium intake, you can easily take a calcium supplement with vitamin D (this vitamin helps to transport and fix the calcium). A healthy body should receive its share of proteins, yet the objective to keep in mind should always be the balanced diet, not forgetting to include a glass of water before eating to reduce hunger pangs, and a glass of water for dessert. Think of water as nature's champagne.

ALCOHOL AND NICOTINE

Alcohol—ethyl alcohol—a stimulant drug at low doses, and a depressant drug at higher doses, is fermented or distilled from sugars and starches to produce C_2H_5OH, the intoxicating agent in beer, wine, whiskey, vodka, gin, tequila, and so on. Normally, when the body communicates desires to the brain, this organ produces chemical signals—neurotransmitters—as a response. These chemical messengers—endorphins, enkephalines, and dopamine—attach to receptors in the brain much like a key fits into a lock. They fill the receptor sites in the reward area, creating a sense of well-being. Alcohol and nicotine target identical cell sites in the nervous system.

When addictive substances like alcohol and nicotine flood the brain, filling the receptors normally occupied by the brain's neurotransmitters, the neurons that normally produce these reward transmitters cut back on their production. The few that are produced are destroyed by the enzyme enkephalinase. After time, because there are more receptor sites and fewer natural neurotransmitters, more of the addictive substance is needed to produce the expected euphoria. Cravings set in, followed by insomnia, depression, and restlessness.

The addiction produced by excessive use of these drugs has three possible sources: a genetic imbalance of neurotransmitters, stress that affects the body's ability to produce neurotransmitters, and chronic substance abuse, which halts the brain's production of neurotransmitters. Chaos erupts in unsatisfied cravings, which lead to a multiplicity of behaviors, all leading to unhappiness. As already noted, Siddhartha revealed that we all desire that which we do not truly desire. Beware of phantom desires.

In the early 1990s it was widely reported that red wine reduced the risk of heart disease. It is currently believed that those who drink in moderation do actually increase their life span. In one study, male heart-attack patients reduced their risks of dying by 28% when they drank 2 to 4 drinks per week. Those who consumed 1 drink per day had a 21% risk, while those who drank 1 to 4 drinks per month had the same reduced risk factor as those who drank 2 or more drinks per day—15%. The optimal level of drinking seems to be one drink per day for men, and about half that for women.

The difference in the tolerance levels between men and women is due to an enzyme in the stomach that breaks down alcohol before it enters the bloodstream—it is four times as active in men as in women. That daily quota of one standard drink is considered to be 12 ounces of beer, 5 ounces of wine, or 1.5 ounces of 80-proof distilled liquor.

Besides the reduced risk of death from coronary heart disease, moderate drinkers enjoyed reduced stress, tension, anxiety, and self-consciousness. For the elderly, moderate drinking stimulates the appetite, promotes proper bowel function, and improves their general mood. Obviously, anyone who has experienced alcohol addiction should try to stay away from any consumption. The potential negative effects far outweigh the possible benefits.

Unfortunately, there are severe side effects to even moderate drinking that increase dramatically as more liquor is consumed. Although blood vessels are less likely to be blocked, strokes are more common, due to bleeding. After just two drinks, the skills of motor coordination, and the perception of time and space necessary for driving a motor vehicle are impaired. Alcohol can interact harmfully with more than 100 medications. With heavier drinkers, certain cancers become more prevalent. Mothers who drink 2 or 3 drinks a day during pregnancy can expect to give birth to smaller babies with a number of minor physical anomalies, and a reduced intelligence as they grow older.

The heavier drinker can expect more misery in his life: car accidents and run-ins with the police, family arguments, violence, and trauma. His body slowly degenerates, provoking: brain damage, cancer, liver disease, pancreatitis, and reproductive failure. Even withdrawal is problematic. Alcohol produces a marked hyperexcitability, hallucinations, insomnia, sleep fragmentation, and tremor. Fortunately, the body can recover. Simply by eating a balanced diet with sufficient amino acids, vitamins, and minerals, neurotransmitters can be regenerated. The real pleasures of normal living can be enjoyed again, although total recovery may take from one to three years. Along the way to that recovery, try a glass of water instead of a drink.   Every time you do, you move one step closer to revitalizing your body and spirit.

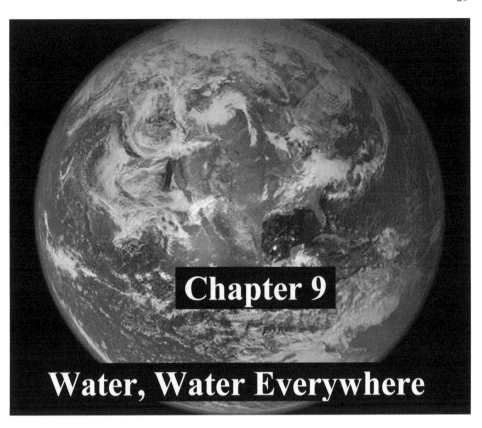

Chapter 9

Water, Water Everywhere

WATER LOSS

Think water. All organic matter on earth is water-based. It is everywhere in us and around us: the clouds, the seas, rivers, lakes, our tears, our bloodstreams, our tissues—it is life itself. An authentic diet must begin at our origins—H_2O. Become conscious of the world you live in. Make it a practice to establish water as your #1 option. Drink a glass of water as soon as you get up. During sleep we lose significant amounts of water by insensible perspiration (i.e., water loss from the skin without sweating), which is the body's mechanism for losing the heat we produce by oxidation. You take a shower, and dry yourself with a towel. Imagine what happens to that wet towel overnight as it dries out. The next morning it is bone dry. Not only does water evaporate from us in the same way, but also sodium and potassium are depleted by constant perspiration. We also breathe out quantities of water vapor along with the carbon dioxide we exhale every few seconds. Fever or hyperventilation can greatly increase this respiratory water loss. The kidneys filter the water from the blood during our sleeping hours, eliminating it the next morning, along with wastes and excess salts. If you choose to stimulate yourself with a morning cup of coffee, do so. But once you have drunk it and, hopefully, eaten a light breakfast, drink a glass of water for dessert. You should feel full, and satisfied.

OUR WATERY NATURE

Because we are a conglomeration of cells whose origins are the oceans, the extracellular fluid that bathes our cells is a saline solution similar to the sea. Once our ancestors left the ocean, they depended on their body's mechanisms to maintain an equilibrium within our internal realm of seawater. The kidneys are the key organs in maintaining that harmony. By controlling the amount of water and plasma constituents the body contains, the kidneys maintain the delicate balance between water and electrolytes that promote good health. When there is an excess of water or an electrolyte such as salt ($NaCl$), the kidneys eliminate the excess in urine. They are extremely flexible doing their job, but even if you do not consume sufficient water, they must still excrete at least a pint of water a day to cleanse the body of wastes.

Water comprises between 40% and 80% of our body weight, depending on the amount of fat (i.e., adipose tissue) an individual has. While fat contains little water (some 10%), plasma consists of more than 90% water. The soft tissues of the body such as skin, muscles, and internal organs are composed of 70% to 80% water. The skeleton is only 22% H_2O. High body water content is related to thinness, while low body water content is related to obesity.

Due to the female sex hormone, estrogen, fat deposits in women's breasts, buttocks, and elsewhere are typical, leading to lower levels of body H_2O. For both men and women, the amount of body water diminishes with age. Body water is distributed between the intracellular fluid found within the cells (two-thirds of the total body H_2O), and the extracellular fluid that surrounds the cells. One-fifth of the extracellular fluid found outside cells is in the liquid part of the blood, plasma. The other four-fifths of the extracellular fluid, tissue fluid, circulates in the spaces around the cells.

The plasma and tissue fluid are separated by the walls of the blood vessels, while the fluids that circulate within and without the cells are separated by the cell walls. The tissue fluid is nearly identical to the plasma, except for the tissue fluid's lack of plasma proteins. These liquids, minus the proteins, are constantly passing through the pores in the thin walls of the capillaries, and mixing. The cells themselves are surrounded by a sensitive plasma membrane that permits the passage of some substances, while denying passage to other substances. All cells are freely permeable to H_2O.

The electrical properties of cells are due to their active transportation of sodium ions out of the cell, and potassium ions into the cell. The water that you drink must first enter the extracellular fluid, and the water that exits the body must also do so via that same extracellular fluid. Proper blood pressure is maintained by the close regulation of the extracellular fluid volume. Salt (NaCl) is the key component in this balancing act. The undesired swelling or shrinking of cells must be controlled by the osmotic actions of the extracellular fluid. (Osmosis is the ability of a solvent to pass through a semi-permeable membrane into a solution of higher concentration in order to equalize the external and internal concentrations.) Cellular water balance is a question of life or death to the body.

Hypertonicity (where water flows out of the cell to dilute the solutes of the cell environment) occurs when there is insufficient water in the system (i.e., dehydration), causing the excessive concentration of solutes outside the cell. Dehydration occurs most often when there is too much water lost by perspiration, vomiting, or diarrhea, or when one suffers from diabetes insipidus. For the vast majority of the population, the solution to this problem is simply to drink sufficient water. And how much is sufficient? Eight glasses a day.

One of the best guarantees of proper water intake is by drinking a glass both during and after each meal, and two other glasses during the day, both as an appetite depressant and as a hydrator. Common symptoms of mild dehydration are dry skin, sunken eyeballs, and less secretion of saliva, resulting in a dry mouth.

Hypotonicity (water flowing into the cell to dilute the solutes within the cell) occurs when there is an abundance of water in the system (i.e., overhydration), causing a dilution in the concentration of solutes. This rarely happens, as the kidneys normally filter out the excess water, which then exits the body via urine.

When there is an imbalance of H_2O, the cells—especially the neurons in the brain—do not function correctly. Any shrinking or swelling must be compensated for immediately by controlling the faulty osmosis due to the overly diluted or overly concentrated extracellular fluid. To maintain a proper balance of water, the amount taken in must equal the amount lost. Typically, we take in 2.6 pints of water in the fluids and foods we consume each day, in addition to 2.1 pints of pure H2O, as well as the metabolic production by our own bodies of an additional 0.7 pints—for a grand total of some 5.5 pints of H2O intake. Our output includes 1.9 pints of insensible loss through breathing and non-sweating skin evaporation, 0.2 pints by sweating, 0.2 pints in our feces, and 3.2 liters via excreted urine—for a grand total of 5.5 pints of H2O loss.

Large amounts of water are contained in the foods we eat. Chicken, fish, and red meat contain about 75% water. Fruits and vegetables vary from 60% to 90% water content. Another often-ignored source of water is found in our own metabolically generated H2O. Food is broken down in our digestive system, and transported to the cells by the liquid river that runs within us. Once delivered by osmosis to the cell, that food is oxidized to release energy, the byproducts being CO2 (carbon dioxide) and H2O. This excess water is absorbed into the extracellular fluid, while the CO2 is transported to the lungs to be breathed out, allowing O2 (oxygen) to be absorbed in the lungs for the return trip to the cell to fuel the slow burning of food.

The volume of extracellular fluid is essential in maintaining proper blood pressure. When the plasma volume is reduced, arterial blood pressure falls. When the plasma volume is increased by an influx of water, the arterial blood pressure rises. There is a constant interplay through the capillary walls in the balance of hydrostatic forces (i.e., the pressure and equilibrium of liquids) and osmotic forces (i.e., when a solvent passes through the semipermeable membrane of the cell wall to equalize concentrations on both sides of the cell wall). When the plasma volume drops, fluid moves out of the interstitial compartment (located between the cellular components of an organ) into the blood vessels, creating an increase in the plasma volume. When the plasma volume is too great, the excess fluid moves into the interstitial compartment. These mechanisms are by nature temporary and limited.

Most important for the long-term blood pressure equilibrium is a proper balance of salt, which controls 90% of the extracellular fluid's osmotic activity. Fresh meat contains more than sufficient salt for our normal needs of half a gram of salt per day, but we are addicted to the taste of salty foods, and therefore consume 10 to 15 grams per day. By allowing ourselves an adequate intake of water, we permit the kidneys to play their key role in blood-pressure maintenance by eliminating the excess salt from our systems via urine. Sweat and feces eliminate the rest. You cannot properly run a water-based system such as ours without adequate water.

EXERCISE

Exercise is necessary for health. Unfortunately, many people feel that more exercise results in greater well-being. They drive themselves beyond normal exercise limits, de-hydrating their bodies and losing excessive amounts of salt. Heat cramps and heat exhaustion can be followed quickly by heat stroke and death. As a result of exercising, large quantities of blood must be pumped to the muscles to provide oxygen and nutriments, while the byproducts in the form of wastes must be removed. These muscles also produce large quantities of heat. The body responds by increasing the blood flow to the skin so that the excess heat can be radiated into the air. If the surrounding air is warmer than the body, no heat can be dissipated through the body's normal cooling system. In fact, the body actually absorbs even more heat from the air. The extra blood that is circulating in the muscles and skin results in less blood returning to the heart. The heart responds by speeding up to deliver the necessary oxygen and nutriments to the muscles, further heating up the body.

During excessive exercise in hot conditions, sweating is increased to cool the body through evaporation. Up to 1.5 liters of water and salts can be lost in an hour of profuse sweating. Without the salt to retain water, the plasma volume is decreased, reducing also the blood supply to the muscles and to the skin for cooling. If excessive exercise continues, the muscles receive the majority of the available blood supply. In an adjustment to keep the cardiac output and blood pressure at proper levels, the skin arterioles become constricted, and are consequently unable to cool the body down. Unless exercise is reduced, body heat rises, the pulse becomes weak, and profuse sweating and disorientation signal heat exhaustion. The temperature control center in the hypothalamus breaks down, and a heat stroke ensues with hot, dry skin, confusion, and unconsciousness, soon followed by death.

Exercising moderately can help one avoid all these unpleasant consequences of overexertion. In some 14 days, the body becomes accustomed to exercising in the heat, and can retain sufficient water to maintain an equilibrium without straining the cardiovascular system. A glass of water should be drunk before exercising, during, and after, and common sense used to limit the stress placed on the body.

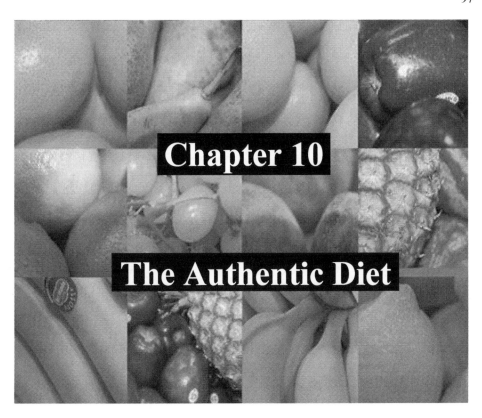

Chapter 10

The Authentic Diet

HEALTH

Let's just assume that the main goal in your pursuit of the authentic diet is primarily focused on good health. As is almost always the case, pursuing the right goal seems to invite desirable secondary effects, like weight loss, higher energy levels, and an enhanced level of spirituality. First, you have to be reasonable, and most of all, honest with yourself. Do you really have sufficient desire and willpower to open your mind to new possibilities, and follow through by establishing sound habits? And can you be shown a way to modify your eating habits to create a new diet that fits you so well, so naturally that it takes no real effort to implement? If you are adverse to chicanery and pain and suffering, then insist on a logical, truthful, natural path to good health. Once you have the mind set, the only way to find out is to try.

We know that the average American's weight is up over 10 pounds since the 1970s. 30% of men and 45% of women do little to no exercise. Some 2 of 3 Americans consume more than 30% of their daily calories in the form of fat. Women typically receive too little zinc, iron, calcium, magnesium, vitamin B6, and vitamin E, while men most typically receive too little magnesium and zinc. Half of all Americans fail to eat even a piece of fruit on any given day. On that same typical day, some 2,200 people are diagnosed with diabetes. And one of the major risk factors for diabetes is being overweight.

OVERWEIGHT?

Obviously, lack of exercise, and overeating the wrong foods contribute to that weight problem. Because eating is a habit, it can be analyzed and modified to better fit our expectancies. Start by taking notes in a diary: what did you eat, and how did you feel after you ate? If you are sleepy or drowsy, you probably consumed too much food and, especially, too many carbohydrates. Make a note of everything that goes into your body, including coffee, tea, liquor, and cigarettes. Review your diary with an especially critical eye on fast-food meals, pizza, chips, cookies, and ice cream—and the time of day they were consumed.

Educate yourself in seconds by reading labels to discover what you are putting into yourself. Exercise a little willpower to deny yourself those fattening, unhealthy snacks, substituting fresh fruits and a glass of water when at all possible. You will feel just as full afterwards, and much more satisfied with yourself. Those cookies, candy bars, popcorn, and ice cream snacks are an illusion—just a trap you get lulled into when you unconsciously reach out for something to satisfy your pangs of hunger and need for fulfillment. Remember Siddhartha's warning about pursuing false desires. Think. Then opt for something more appropriate. Would you fill your gas tank with kerosene or diesel oil before heading out on a trip?

Make a concerted effort to stop buying donuts, candies, ice cream, and junk food. Simply do not have them at home! Make a list of appetizing fruits and vegetables, and then shop in your local supermarket with some imagination and determination. Most of that incredible selection of fresh fruits and vegetables has been harvested and transported hundreds of miles from your home, and delivered virtually to your doorstep. Open your mind to the possibilities. At home, condition yourself to take the few seconds necessary to slice up some fresh fruits and vegetables, and serve them as snacks and dessert.

Cook and serve green vegetables on a daily basis. Serve everyone a sampling, and encourage their consumption. Be determined to seek a healthy path by eating sound foods, but do so gradually, consistently elevating the level of your family's diet. Begin to watch your calorie intake. Get up and take a refreshing walk. And maintain a safe distance from fad diets. They will entice you with quick answers; you will lose weight initially with any of them, suffer some, then regain all, if not more of the pounds you painfully shed.

Now is the time indicated to begin creating a well-balanced diet of sufficient amounts of proteins, lipids (fats and other substances with similar properties), carbohydrates, vitamins and minerals. Adopting a diet that fits your particular needs and tastes, reduces the risk of cardiovascular diseases, diabetes, cancer, colds, infections, and so on. Digestive irregularities like diarrhea and constipation are also reduced. Obesity becomes easier to control. Is it any wonder a good diet produces good feelings?

SCHEDULE

Meals should be enjoyed at regular hours. Never skip a meal. Take your time to make the meal a pleasurable experience: chew the pleasure out of each mouthful. Vary your diet to avoid boredom. Eat sufficient amounts of carbohydrates, dairy products, meat, fish, eggs, vegetables, and fruits. Minimize the amount of fats hidden in pastries, dressings, and sauces.

Drink a glass of water during each meal, and one after. When those irresistible hunger pangs gnaw at you between meals, pick up a fresh fruit, and follow it with a sparkling glass of water. Then pat yourself on the back for making such a wise choice. Be conscious of your decisions. These wise choices become habits that create a healthier you.

Try eating four small meals a day. Include in each a lean portion of protein in the form of fish, chicken (without the skin), lean meat, or beans. To complete the well-rounded meal, add a portion of vegetables or fruit. (A portion is about the size of a chicken leg, a piece of fruit, or half a cup of rice or beans.) By avoiding fatty foods, and eating a diet with larger amounts of high-fiber foods, diarrhea and constipation can be more easily controlled. Unfortunately, if you attempt to shift your diet too quickly to high concentrations of fiber, cramping and intestinal gas will often accompany the change. Learn your habits by careful observation, noting them in a diary format, then gradually change course. Old habits cannot be undone overnight.

EGGS

Eggs are included in the protein group, but no one seems to know how many can be safely consumed. The American Heart Association and the National Institutes of Health have set the limit at 3 to 4 eggs per week, but recent research indicates that up to 2 eggs a day can be eaten without flooding the cardiovascular system with excessive cholesterol.

VEGETABLES

The most beneficial of the green vegetables is the dark-green variety, such as: arugula, beet greens, bok choy, cabbage, chard, collard greens, kale, mustard greens, radicchio, rapini, and turnip greens. They are good sources of phytochemicals, elements that seem to reduce the risk of heart disease. Furthermore, they contain no fats nor cholesterol, and yield only 5-20 calories per serving. They are rich in the antioxidants vitamins A and C, and beta-carotene. These antioxidants reduce the amount of free radicals, which are produced by normal body processes like breathing, yet are highly destructive. The consumption of alcohol, the smoking of cigarettes, and the breathing of polluted air also increase the body's levels of free radicals. By consuming high amounts of green vegetables, fruits, whole grains, and legumes, you reduce the risks from heart disease, as well as other afflictions, such as cancer.

FIBER

Fiber is the plant cell-wall material, and internal structures of foods like vegetables, fruits, and whole grains. It is believed to reduce the risk of heart disease, high blood pressure, cancer, and obesity. Fresh fruits high in fiber are apples, oranges, and pears. Fresh vegetables high in fiber are broccoli, cabbage, cauliflower, lima beans, and spinach. Dried beans are also a good source for fiber, especially chickpeas and kidney beans. Fiber is easily obtainable, yet Americans manage to eat only half the recommended 25-35 grams per day.

FOLATE

The folate that is found in raw leafy vegetables helps reduce the amino acid homocysteine found in the blood. This amino acid is linked to heart disease. Unfortunately, cooking eliminates 50% of the folate from vegetables. They are better used in raw salads. If you choose to cook the dark-green vegetables, try microwaving them to retain their nutrients. They can also be sautéed with a splash of olive oil. Steaming greens also retains much of their nutritional value. They can be seasoned with garlic, lemon, olive oil, or soy sauce.

PHYTOCHEMICALS

Phytochemicals are compounds produced by plants to ward off bacteria, fungi, and viruses. Among some 600 already identified, is aresaponins, a class of phytochemicals found in alfalfa sprouts, legumes (i.e., dry beans and peas), oats, potatoes, spinach, and tomatoes. Besides defending the plant from invasion, they protect our bodies from some kinds of tumor cells, especially lung and blood cancers, by interfering with their DNA replication. Saponins have also been found to lower blood cholesterol by inhibiting its absorption in the small intestine, or inhibiting the reabsorption of bile acids.

Another family of phytochemicals is isoflavones, found in soybeans, and in lesser amounts in garbanzo beans. By mimicking the action of estradiol, a naturally occurring estrogen, they help prevent heart disease by reducing the blood level of cholesterol. Research indicates they have antioxidant properties, preventing the smooth muscle cells that line the arteries from clumping together to form part of the plaque build up, while also helping prevent blood clots, and maintaining blood vessel walls elastic and resilient.

CANCER

The World Cancer Research Fund and the American Institute for Cancer Research recommend 5 to 10 servings of fruits and vegetables a day to prevent cancer. Foods found to deter up to 20% of all incidents of cancer include the vegetables from the cabbage family: broccoli, Brussels sprouts, cauliflower, and kale. Also effective are dried beans and peas, tomatoes, deep yellow-orange vegetables and fruits, citrus fruits, blueberries, and dried fruits like prunes and raisins.

Citrus juices, especially orange and tangerine, have been found to contain 22 substances called flavonoids. Two flavonoids found in tangerine juice, tangeretin and nobiletin, are effective in inhibiting the growth of prostate cancer cells. Another flavonoid found in both tangerines and oranges, 5-desmethyl sinensetin, has proven effective in inhibiting the growth of cancer cells in the lungs.

FATS

The reason too many Americans are obese today is not due to the fats we consume, but more specifically to the huge amounts of calories we gobble down, and the lack of exercise to burn them off. In fact, fats supply us with vitamins A, D, E, and K. Many fats serve us well: milk fat contains anti-cancer substances like conjugated linoleic acid. Vegetable oils and fish supply us with polyunsaturated fatty acids, liquid at room temperature. They are found in corn, safflower, sesame, and sunflower oils, which in turn are mixed into salad dressing, mayonnaise, and margarine. Gizzards and giblets have a low fat content, but are high in cholesterol. Omega-3 poly-unsaturated fatty acids are derived from fish. Sources for monounsaturated fats are avocados and nuts, as well as canola (rapeseed), olive, and peanut oil. Monounsaturated and polyunsaturated fats do not contribute to serum cholesterol or low-density lipoprotein (LDL) levels, and seem to reduce heart disease risk.

Saturated fats raise the blood cholesterol levels, promoting plaque formation. These fats are solid at room temperature. They are naturally occurring animal fats, but can also be formed by hydrogenation (i.e., combined with hydrogen) of unsaturated vegetable oil. Hydrogenated fats are used to increase the shelf life of foods like cookies, crackers, doughnuts, French fries, and potato chips. These animal and plant fats also contribute to heart disease. The typical American consumes some 15% of these fats in his diet. The outstanding culprits are: chicken fat (30%), vegetable shortening (31%), lard (40%), beef fat (50%), butter (62%), palm kernel oil (81%), and coconut oil (86%).

RED MEAT AND FISH

Consumption of red meat should be limited to 6 ounces a day—about the size of a large hamburger. When shopping for beef, try to cut down on the fat content by buying "select" cuts.

Beef labeled "choice" is moderately high in fat content, but more desirable than the fat-laden "prime" cuts. Beef consumption can be greatly reduced by building it into a well-balanced meal.

The more fish you eat, the less likely you are to suffer from a stroke. Cold-water fish like mackerel, salmon, trout, and tuna contain omega-3 fatty acids that prevent blood platelets from clotting and sticking to blood vessel walls. Since blood clots cause 80% of strokes, eating fish 5 times per week has been shown to reduce the risk of strokes by over 50%. Eating fish 2 to 4 times per week reduces stroke risk by over 25%. High doses of omega-3 fatty acids can also reduce blood pressure. For maximum benefit, fish should be broiled or baked, not fried.

NUTS

In small amounts, nuts can add variety to your diet. They contain fat, but mostly unsaturated fat, which can actually act to lower the low-density lipoproteins (i.e., the "bad" cholesterol, LDL). The antioxidants in nuts can aid the immune system combat heart disease and cancer. Again, moderation is the key to enjoying this food. The soybean is a member of the pea family, and contains quantities of protein and oil. Not only has it proven itself useful in preventing heart disease, but also seems to combat cancer, menopausal symptoms, and osteoporosis. Soy can be used in a multitude of dishes as tofu, but also can be used as nuts in salads, and drunk as soy milk. We will hear much more from the mighty soybean in the future.

LABELS

Food labels give us essential information about the amount of fat, cholesterol, fiber, calories, and sodium that foods contain. Each gram of fat contains 9 calories, while proteins and carbohydrates each contain 4 calories per gram (1 ounce = 28.35 grams). The Food and Drug Administration recommends a ceiling of fat calories at 30% of our total intake. That represents 600 fat calories (65 grams) for a typical female adult with a consumption of 2,000 calories per day, and 750 fat calories (80 grams) for a typical male adult with a consumption of 2,500 calories per day. Of that total, a maximum of 20 grams for females and 25 grams for males should be saturated fats.

By taking the time to read labels, it should be easy enough to stay within the limits of 2,400 milligrams of sodium per day. Cholesterol should be limited to 300 milligrams per day. Vitamins A, C, E, and calcium are generally found on the product's label. A fiber intake of 25 grams per day can also be monitored from a quick look at labels. Products labeled as "low fat" must contain fewer than 3 grams of fat per serving. Beware of deceptive advertising of products high in carbohydrates passing themselves off as low in fats and cholesterol. The more interested you are in your own health, and that of your family, the more educated you become, and the easier it becomes to focus on healthy foods.

THE DIET PLAN

Common sense and a little concrete knowledge come into play when planning your diet strategy. Forget about fad diets and magic potions that promise you heaven. They allow you to shed water, yet soon leave you disillusioned and disgusted with yourself. Establish a strategy based on solid dietary facts. Create meal plans and grocery lists based on sound science and your real needs. Record your food intake in a sketchy diary, take a good look at your eating behavior, and analyze your habits with the intent of modifying them, to put them into harmony with your body's demands.

Once you have a plan in mind, take one small step at a time. Rid your house of junk food, and stock up on fruits and other sound nutriments—and especially, do not forget the water. Buy a variety of water, from mineral-laden to bubbly, and place it where it will remind you just how inviting it is. Pour it into a champagne glass, serve it on the rocks, think of it as the cool nectar from a fresh mountain stream, as the sparkling fountain in a desert oasis.

Get out of the habit of reaching for the first mouthful of food that appeals to you. With a minimum of effort, plan your meals. Measure the portions. You tend to eat what is placed before you, so be less spontaneous, and think out your meal strategy. 30% of us eat out at any given meal, so eat modestly of buffets, junk food, greasy cheeseburgers and fries, chocolate malts, and all the other food substitutes that are really mirages, the false desires that leave us empty and disillusioned. Drink a glass of water before you sit down to eat—and drink it with pleasure. Water is the essence of life. Do not skip breakfast. Keep to a schedule when you can count on eating meals regularly. Serve yourself on a small plate to make your meal appear plentiful. Eat slowly, with gusto. Enjoy the variety nature has provided us.

Get in touch with yourself. True "hunger" is both a biological and physiological response of the brain and body to the need for nourishment. Real hunger evokes stomach pangs, intestinal rumblings, or a headache. On the other hand, "appetite" is a psychological response to external stimuli ranging from magazine and TV advertisements to mental images and emotional habits—dancing visions intended to satisfy emotional ups and downs, responses to a world of inviting images. We all know not to shop for food when we are hungry. Keep snacks out of sight or, better yet, get rid of them. When food cues like movie popcorn, cake-and-ice cream billboards, and fast-food arches penetrate your senses, wake up and ask yourself some key questions. When did I last eat? What am I really craving? Is my hunger internal or external? What is causing my desire?

Think ahead. Make a plan to deal with those over-whelming cravings, and take command of yourself. You can make it easier if you substitute fresh fruits and a glass of water for those false desires, and soon you should realize that you have made a habit of sound nutrition. We all have our demons, yet when we confront them, we discover they are made of nothing more than papier-maché.

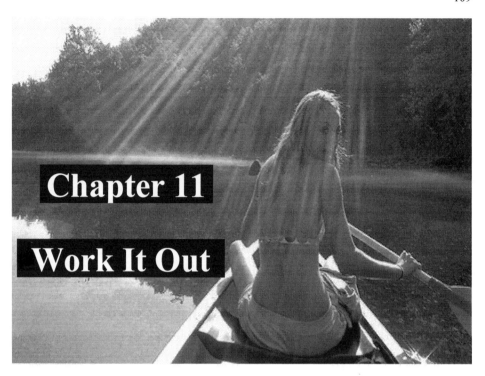

Chapter 11
Work It Out

BENEFITS

Exercise: the systematic practice of an activity for training or developing the mind and body. The fundamental concept seems to dwell in "systematic." Not only does a successful exercise plan involve carefully choosing a series of activities that promote good health, yet are appropriate to your particular situation, and mental and physical state, but also one that can naturally become habitual. Basically, to live on Planet Earth means to exercise just to get about. Here we will be talking about exercising to slightly exceed the demands of common locomotion, therefore creating a comfort zone during normal activities. Consider trying to reserve a little time every day to exercise for fun, and for the dramatic results it can bring in your health and spirit. It really can be pleasurable.

Just existing—the obstinate refusal to engage in any physical activity beyond the merely essential, leads not only to obesity, but also results in high blood pressure, a low level of high-density lipoproteins (HDL—the "good" cholesterol), and diabetes. By attempting to moderately condition our bodies, we should expect an improved flexibility, some buildup of muscular strength, and an increased endurance. Compared to an inactive person's heart rate of 70 to 75 beats per minute, a well-conditioned person's heart beats 45 to 50 times in that same minute. In a day, that adds up to 36,000 fewer heartbeats, and in a year, a staggering 13 million fewer beats. Exercise also results in a marked increase in bone and muscle mass, and stronger joints. Incidences of a variety of illness and diseases are reduced, including colon cancer and strokes. There is a notable improvement in mood, with a reduced sense of depression and anxiety.

One study revealed that people who had exercised and subsequently quit, experienced depression at a rate of 1.5 times that of those who continued exercising. Active people can expect to be better adjusted, experience a higher level of mental activity, and suffer less from stress, anxiety, and depression. They generally feel more self-confidence and higher self-esteem than those who choose not to maintain an active life-style. Working out is an avenue for eliminating those feelings of hopelessness, nervousness, sadness, and worthlessness. Exercise also induces the body to create healthier bone mass and muscles, and more resilient joints. It has even been shown that those people who smoke and exercise tend to reduce the amount of smoking they engage in.

It seems all too obvious that a healthy body and spirit are directly linked to a regimen of exercise. The principal variables in a serious effort at an exercise regimen include the frequency that we perform the exercises, the intensity that we perform them, and the duration of the actual exercises. Each of us has his own formula, which can be modified to adapt to our individual needs and goals.

GETTING IT DONE

Make your exercise agenda a positive experience by coming prepared. (1) Purchase a comfortable pair of workout shoes. (2) Select music you enjoy to work out with. (3) Come with a positive attitude. (4) Wear comfortable clothing. (5) Drink water before, during, and after working out. (6) Women should buy a quality sports bra. (7) Use safe, quality equipment. (8) Use gloves when appropriate. (9) Schedule sufficient time. (10) Find a workout partner if desired. (11) Seek fresh, clean air, and sunshine. (12) Make a plan, keep an exercise diary, modify it as necessary, but stick to it.

Highly productive exercises include brisk walking, stair climbing, jogging, running, hiking, bicycling, swimming, rowing, and sports like soccer, basketball, tennis, racquetball, and touch football. Such aerobic exercises condition the heart and lungs by increasing the efficiency of oxygen intake by the body. For maximum benefit, these activities should be carried out for 30-60 minutes at a time, at least 3 to 4 days per week, at an intensity of 50-75% of your maximum heart rate. Obviously, a real effort must be made to schedule these activities, and realize them with consistency.

If this level of exercising seems like an overwhelming burden, other options are readily available. Above all, ease into an exercise program adapted to your own entry level and overall goals. There is no rush. Create a sensible program, and be ready to adapt it. If you experience any adverse physical symptoms, consult your doctor without hesitation. People who know or suspect they have cardiovascular, metabolic, neurological, orthopedic, or respiratory disorders must consult their doctors before beginning or modifying their exercise plans.

YOUR HEART

A healthy reminder: every year in the United States nearly 1.5 million Americans suffer a heart attack. Of those, half a million die. Coronary heart disease is the number 1 killer and disabler in our country. Every 20 seconds, a heart attack strikes another victim. The only proven way out of this dilemma is by a serious change in lifestyle. Knowing that the three primary risk factors are high blood pressure, high blood cholesterol, and cigarette smoking, one should feel compelled to make a major shift in life style by confronting these issues face to face, and resolving a plan to minimize their effects.

We do know that heart disease is about twice as likely in inactive people. Fatty deposits build up on the inner walls of the coronary arteries and can either starve the heart muscle by blocking its blood flow, or stop up the blood flow to the heart muscle by a blood clot. High blood pressure is indicated when it exceeds 140/90 mmHg (i.e., millimeters of mercury). High blood cholesterol is defined as exceeding 240 mg/dl (i.e., milligrams per deciliter). Smokers are 2 to 4 times more likely to suffer a heart attack.

BENEFITS

The secondary effects of improved health include reduced absenteeism, accidents, and healthcare costs, including rehabilitation. A little exercise is a good start; cutting back or eliminating smoking is a major step; and developing a sound diet plan is the last key element. Of course, reducing stress and other threatening factors can prove to be lifesaving as well. And to think that the first tiny step might simply consist of a toast to our new awareness and resolve with a fresh glass of sparkling water.

Not only should general health and psychological concerns motivate you, but also you should expect an improved self-image, a marked resistance to fatigue, and an improved ability not only to fall asleep quickly, but also to sleep the whole night through. Look for ways to share your activity with friends or family.

BURNING CALORIES

In order to lose 1 pound of fat, you must burn off 3,500 calories. Of course, the less you weigh, the fewer calories you naturally burn off. In the normal course of events, you burn approximately 75% of your daily energy by simply breathing, digesting food, sitting, and sleeping. The following is a list of activities, and the amount of calories burned by a typical 150-pound individual.

Activity	Calories/Hour Burned
bicycling 6 m/hr	240
bicycling 12 m/hr	410
walking 2 m/hr	240
walking 3 m/hr	320
walking 4 ½ m/hr	440
jogging 5 ½ m/hr	740
jogging 7 m/hr	920

running in place 1 hr	650
running 10 m/hr	1280
swimming 25 yds/min	275
swimming 50 yds/min	500
tennis	400

LISTEN TO YOUR BODY

Do not overdo it. If you begin too hard, or exercise for too long, you risk injury to your muscles and joints. Also, on hot days, drink plenty of water before, during, and after exercising. Be aware of the symptoms of heat exhaustion: confusion, dizziness, headache, nausea, and a high body temperature. If you fail to care for yourself, heat exhaustion can potentially lead to heat stroke, further involving: muscle cramps, the complete stopping of sweating, and a high body temperature. Use common sense, and listen to your body's signals. If you ever experience chest pain, dizziness, fainting, or extreme breathlessness, visit your doctor immediately.

For those who do not wish to engage in such demanding activities, low-intensity exercises can benefit them by engaging the body from 40% to 60% of its maximum capacity. This level of exercising includes dancing, housework, gardening, and walking for pleasure. The object is to occupy the large muscles in continuous activity for 30 to 60 minutes, 3 to 6 times a week.

WARM-UP

As is always the case before exercising, warm up. Loosen

up the arms, chest, back, and leg muscles by following a routine similar to the following. Roll your head in five 360-degree turns, and then reverse the direction for another five turns. Extend your arms straight out, and then roll them like windmills five times in giant arcs. Reverse direction for another set of rolls. Rotate the shoulders in five forward loop shrugs, and then reverse them. Rotate your trunk five times around your waist, and then reverse the rotation for an additional five turns.

Keeping the back straight, do five knee bends. Keep within your comfort range. Standing, extend one leg slightly, make it limp, then shake it; then extend the other and shake it. Stretch your arms upward, then sweep forward, downward, then backward. Reverse direction. Extend your arms limply, and then shake them out. Clench, and then unclench your fists ten times. Repeat any of the above limbering exercises as desired.

USE A CHAIR

Sit in a comfortable chair with armrests. Raise your arms high in the air, and dip your torso down to one side, rise up, and then continue dipping down and rising up in a semicircle until you have rotated as far as comfortable. Reverse direction and repeat. Place your fists together before your chest, and then stretch your elbows backward. Flap like a chicken. Do another set of head rolls. Lift your feet off the ground, and then replace them. Now stand behind your chair, grasp the back for support, and do five knee lifts with each leg. Repeat, further away from your body. Next, extend your leg straight, and then lift. Rotate it clockwise, and then counter-clock-wise in large circles. Repeat with the other leg. Follow this by five shallow knee bends. Keep your back straight, and do not bend the knees too deeply. Now lift your leg backwards five times in a soft, swinging motion. Stretch yourself like a cat. Repeat as desired.

Step away from the chair, and run in place for 30 seconds. Grasp the back of the chair again, and rise up on your toes without bouncing, and then return your heels to the floor. Repeat five times.

Sit in your chair, and with your back straight, grasp the arms of the chair and push yourself upwards according to your own ability to do so. Stand, extend your arms with palms down, and clench and unclench your fists five times. Do the same with your palms facing upwards. Now do the same with your arms extended straight up into the air. Repeat this entire series of clenches, but this time with added strength. You might choose to grasp a tennis ball in each hand. Next, use one hand to stretch the fingers of your other hand upwards, and then downwards, simply to loosen them up. Rotate your wrists as you move your clenched fists in tight circles.

Stand a short distance from the wall, and lean against it with your palms. Place one foot forward, and one back. Stretch the calf on the back leg, but do not bounce. Switch legs and repeat.

Sit down again, grasp the armrests, and lean forward as if to tie your shoelaces. Keeping your feet flat on the floor, try to stretch the back and hamstring muscles as you bend over, and then sit back upright. Now stand and stretch your legs out. Shake them. Next, grasp the armrests, and bend toward the chair seat. The object is just to loosen up the leg and back muscles. Now spread the legs wider, and shift weight over the hips from one leg to the other, trying to stretch the inner thigh muscles. Stretch and shake them out when satisfied you have done enough. Easy does it.

ON YOUR BACK

To work on the abdominal area, lie down on your back on a soft surface. Hold your knees to your chest, and then rock from side to side. Next, lie down flat on your back, placing your hands on your thighs, then rise up slightly in a partial sit-up. The lifting motion alone will condition the abdomen. Shift your hands to behind your head and lock the fingers together, and then do another short series of lifts, assuring that the focus be on the abdomen.

If you experience cramping or discomfort, a gentle pounding of the fists on the stomach area should relieve the tension of the muscles. Again, from a position flat on your back, and grasping your hands behind your head, lift one knee up to your chest, moving the opposite elbow toward the knee. Repeat some five times, then do the same on the opposite side.

From the same position flat on your back, place your palms beneath your buttocks, and lift both knees up to your chest. Lower them. Repeat five times. It is never necessary to strain in an attempt to go beyond the natural limits of your body. In this instance, the mere effort to reach your chest is sufficient to realize the objectives of this exercise.

HEARTBEAT

Your target heart-rate zone should be from 50% to 75% of your maximum rate. That maximum rate per minute is about 220, minus your age. To determine your heartbeats per minute, take your pulse as soon as you stop exercising. Do so by placing the tips of your fingers lightly over the carotid arteries in your neck (located on either side of your Adam's apple), or by placing your fingertips inside your wrist just below the base of your thumb. Count the pulses for 10 seconds, and then multiply by 6. The following is a table of heartbeats for various ages.

Age	Target Heartbeats/Min. Maximum	Normal Heartbeat
20	100-150	200
25	98-146	195
30	95-142	190
35	93-138	185
40	90-135	180
45	88-131	175
50	85-127	170
55	83-123	165
60	80-120	160
65	78-116	155
70	75-113	150

WEIGHT TRAINING

Of the four components of fitness: aerobic exercise, flexibility, diet, and resistance, the latter—weight training—can make the greatest difference. For an individual of any age, it redefines the body, allowing for more mobility and balance. It has been shown to maintain bone density. Just lifting weights twice a week for four months increases the utilization of glucose by nearly 25%, reducing the risk of diabetes. "Good" HDL (high-density lipoproteins) are increased, while "bad" LDL (low-density lipoproteins) are decreased. Blood pressure is lowered. Depression is diminished.

Even though we lose muscle mass as we age, there is no time limit on becoming involved with weights. Research at Ohio State University revealed that men between 60 and 75 are able to increase their strength by 50% to 80% in four months. At Boston's Tufts University, a group of 90-year-olds improved their strength by nearly 175% after eight weeks of weight training.

At the University of Alabama, a group of men and women ranging in age from 61 to 77 lost an average of 6 pounds of fat, while gaining 4.5 pounds of muscle in a strength-training program that met three times a week for six months. Their bodies burned an extra 230 calories a day compared to what they had burned at the beginning of weight training—whether they exercised that day or not.

When weights are lifted, micro tears in the muscles occur, which cause the body to begin repairing itself, further building muscle mass. With more muscle mass, more calories are needed to keep the added muscles nourished. The result is more body fat being burned up to supply the energy demanded by the new muscles and their heightened activity. And even more body fat can be eliminated if a regular weight-training program is combined with aerobic exercises.

Women do not bulk up as was once popularly believed. In fact, by lifting weights, women have the added benefit of reducing the risk for osteoporosis, as well as gaining a more attractive shape. Besides improved bone density, females achieve an increase in energy levels, and discover a diminishing of their overall weight. For women as for men, a continued regimen of resistance training promises vibrancy in the advancing years, instead of the normal sense of inevitable decline.

Strength training normally means employing up to 10 exercise sets to target various muscle groups: arms, shoulders, chest, trunk, hips, legs, and back. Each set should involve moderate weights with 10 to 15 repetitions, a minimum of twice weekly. Although the weights are moderate (5-10 pound dumbbells are sufficient), you need to push yourself to make a significant difference. By exhausting the muscles, you are actually promoting muscle rebuilding and reconditioning.

In overloading the muscles, aim for a lifting weight of 60% to 80% of what you determine to be your maximum lift. You should never feel pain, although it is common to experience soreness, especially on the second day after your workout. This soreness, however, is the natural byproduct of the body's effort to eliminate waste products and toxins produced within the working muscles.

TECHNIQUE

Performing the weight lifting properly is essential. Weights are meant to target certain muscle groups and give them a thorough working out. You should never use the natural momentum or swing of your body, but rather isolate and expose the target muscle groups to as strenuous an exercise as you feel reasonable. Your goal should be to overload all your muscle groups in any given session, always seeking variety in speed of execution and order. Consult a certified trainer or qualified instructor to assure you of proper technique and weight limits. Overall, this should be an enjoyable activity that has the potential to quickly improve your quality of life.

Select a pair of dumbbells that fit your needs—5 pounds each should be sufficient. You should be able to do 5-10 repetitions at a time with them, but they should weigh enough to take you to your endurance limits. Stretch your body with warm-up exercises. Begin with neck rolls, arm rolls and flaps, then move on to waist rolls, half-knee bends, then toe touches, periodically shaking out the stretched muscles.

Once you feel loose enough, go through your short program of lifting. Try to accomplish more by repetition and "exploding" (often "exploding" is more of a motivational term, not to be taken literally) than by methodical lifting of heavy weights. Sample the following exercises, and then develop your own routine by selecting the most practical and beneficial ones for yourself. Invent, borrow, and adapt to create your unique repertoire.

1. Standing with dumbbells hanging from your arms, lift them straight upward and forward until your arms are parallel with the ground, then lower your arms.

2. Do #1 again, this time beginning by rotating the palms outward.

3. Repeat #1 and #2, but lifting straight in front of yourself, with the dumbbells nearly touching.

4. With the dumbbells hanging from your arms, do a half-squat. From the down position, bounce back to upright. Keep your back straight.

5. Keeping your back straight, either pick the dumbbells up from the floor, or begin as low as you can. Lift them straight up, rotate your wrists until they are on level with your chin, and then explode them as high as you can above your head. Slowly lower them as close to the floor as you can.

6. Lie on your back, your elbows on the floor, arms pointed upwards, dumbbells in hands. Explode the weights upwards to full arm extension, and then lower them slowly to vertical rest.

7. Begin by lying on your back with your arms flat on the floor, dumbbells in hands, arms extended straight out to form a cross. Bring your arms up to vertical, then down to rest on the floor. Do the same with your arms extended above your head.

8. Place your knee and one arm on a chair or bench. Suspend a dumbbell from the free hand, bring it straight up to your side, and then lower it. Change hands.

PREPARATION

Prepare before you exercise. Avoid injuries to feet, ankles, legs and joints by never pushing yourself too far, too soon. Know when to rest. Wear clothing that is appropriate for the exercise. On warm days, that means light, loose-fitting clothing. On cold days, use gloves and several layers of clothing, yet one layer less than you would if you were not exercising. Because some 40% of our body heat is radiated from our heads and necks, wear a hat. If you have just eaten, wait 2 hours before working out. After your workout, wait at least 20 minutes before eating. Try to stay away from hard surfaces such as sidewalks and concrete courts. If running on roadways, wear clothing that is easily visible, and run against traffic. When riding bicycles, use a helmet, and avoid busy streets. Shopping malls make ideal all-weather walking tracks, and can be entertaining and socializing as well.

WALKING AND JOGGING

A fruitful walking program can begin with a 5-minute stroll, followed by a brisk 7-minute walk, then another 5-minute stroll. Try this 3 times the first week, then each succeeding week increase the brisk walk by 2 minutes. Check your pulse periodically to see if you fall within your target zone. Keep a record. If you wish to jog, begin with a 5-minute walk followed by some stretching exercises, and then a 5-minute brisk walk, followed by a 1-minute jog. Walk it off for 3 minutes, and then stretch for 2 minutes. Be sure to record your pulse rate at regular intervals. Each week you can increase the jogging segment by 2 minutes. Drink a glass of water before you begin your workout, and another glass after you finish. Avoid sodas, cigarettes, and alcohol as best as you can. As you begin to reclaim your health, you will be amazed at how good you feel.

CUSTOMIZING

Even before you begin an exercise program, determine how physically fit you are at the moment. Do not be in a hurry. Always begin with less-vigorous activities, and build up to more-demanding ones. Consider your age. Have a concrete idea of the benefits you should expect. Once you have written down short-term and long-term goals, discuss them with a friend or family member. Keep an accurate record of your achievements and progress. Determine whether you prefer group activities, exercising with a partner, or alone. If you are bored with an activity, vary or replace it. Know the money parameters of your desired activities. Factor in convenience, feasibility, and desirability when you are creating a schedule. Commit to a long-term plan, yet always remain flexible to allow for unforeseen elements.

Create a new awareness of yourself, your health needs, and the world you live in. Consider choosing stairs as a viable alternative to riding the elevator. Park a comfortable walking distance from work or shopping. Create activity breaks to get up, stretch, and move around. Instead of filling yourself up with junk food, choose to take a brief walk instead, and relish a tall glass of cool water to quench that desire to snack.

Up the ante—when you perform any mundane physical task, like housework, do it with vigor. Pull yourself away from the TV or computer to run your own errands, empty the garbage, mow the lawn, carry your groceries, walk the dog—all with the intent of getting a healthy workout in the process. And never forget that key element in any healthy activity—water!

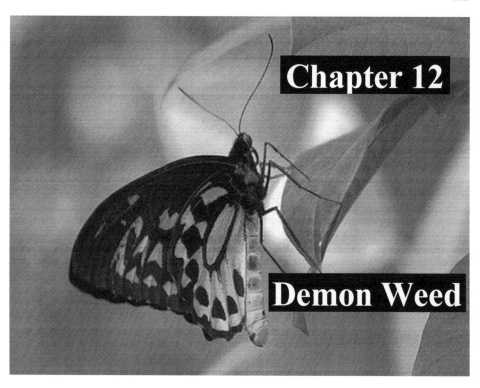

Chapter 12

Demon Weed

THE HISTORY OF TOBACCO

Some 20,000 years ago, towards the end of the last ice age, nomadic tribes from Manchuria followed migrating game across the land bridge of the Bering Strait from what is now Russia into Alaska. They continued wandering in small groups until they had populated the Americas. By 11,000 B.C. some of these Paleoindians had made their way onto the lowlands of Patagonia, the Pampas, and Gran Chaco in South America, where they found wild tobacco growing abundantly. It would be another 3,000 years until they began experiencing the benefits of agriculture, and started cultivating tobacco in their gardens.

This tropical plant of the nightshade family has hairy, sticky foliage that contains an abundance of a poisonous, water-soluble alkaloid, $C_{10}H_{14}N_2$—nicotine, named after Jean Nicot, the French ambassador at Lisbon who first introduced tobacco to France in 1560. These indigenous peoples grew 12 different species of tobacco, most noteworthy being the *Nicotiana tabacum* and *Nicotiana rustica*.

Tobacco soon became an ingrained element of their culture. Not only would they smoke great quantities of it on ceremonial occasions, but they would also snuff it, chew it, drink its juice and syrup, lick a paste of tobacco, and give tobacco enemas. It was used topically on the skin and the eyes. In its ritual use, the shamans were known to smoke one huge 3-foot cigar after another, attempting to intoxicate themselves to the brink of death, expecting in that way to gain spiritual insights into the origins and true nature of diseases. The pure potency of the native tobacco and the great amounts they inhaled induced hallucinations. Filling the air and their lungs with great clouds of smoke, the shamans attempted to bridge the gap between the material and the spiritual worlds. Thousands of years later, we are still intoxicating our minds and disorienting our spirits with this obnoxious weed.

When Christopher Columbus first set foot in the New World on San Salvador Island in 1492, the indigenous Arawaks brought him gifts of fruit, wooden spears, and dried tobacco leaves. Once back on board his ship, Columbus sampled the fruit, and discretely tossed the fragrant tobacco leaves overboard. Good riddance. In the same year, Rodrigo de Jerez stopped in Cuba on his search for the passage to China. There he observed natives tightly wrapping dried tobacco leaves in cornhusks, lighting one end, then "drinking" the smoke through the other end. Jerez was soon caught up in this exotic ritual, and brought back to Spain a considerable store of tobacco to feed his habit. When his neighbors caught sight of the smoke billowing out of his nose and mouth, he was reported to the Holy Inquisitors, and subsequently imprisoned for 7 years. By the time he regained his freedom, Spaniards were enthusiastically smoking tobacco throughout the kingdom.

When Europeans first made contact with the Haida Indians of the Queen Charlotte Islands off the west coast of Canada, and the Tlingit Indians on the southern coast of Alaska, they found them chewing tobacco. Both groups of natives had environments so plentiful and varied in food sources, they had no need to develop agricultural techniques—except to grow tobacco. It is postulated that many such societies converted from their traditional hunting and gathering to a sedentary lifestyle based on agriculture in order to guarantee for themselves a constant supply of tobacco.

The Haida would plant their seeds towards the end of April, inserting one pod into a mound of earth. The plants were cared for until September, when the tobacco leaves were harvested. Their harvest was then dried on a wooden frame over a fire. Once dried, the leaves were ground with a mortar and pestle. Burnt shells were ground and added as a lime catalyst to the center of the plug of tobacco to be chewed.

When Hernán Cortés first visited the Aztec capital in Mexico in 1519, he saw perfumed reed cigarettes being sold in the market square. By 1531, Europeans were cultivating tobacco in Santo Domingo, and by 1534, "tall tobacco," the sweet, broadleaved *Nicotiana tabacum* was brought from Central America to be cultivated in Cuba. The Portuguese had established tobacco plantations in Brazil by 1548. Soon Europe was inebriated by the drug. In 1560, Jean Nicot (Mr. Nicotine himself) was proclaiming the medicinal properties of tobacco, labeling it a panacea. When he gave some snuff to Catherine de Medici, Queen of France, to treat her son's migraine headaches, she declared it "Herba Regina."

In 1564 Sir John Hawkins introduced tobacco to England. In Spain, tobacco was termed a miracle drug, able to cure some 36 maladies. By the 17th century, tobacco had become the monetary standard in the American Colonies. In fact, this cash crop replaced the gold standard during the 17th and 18th centuries. It became the source of wealth in the middle Southern States, and the standard value against which all merchandise was measured.

EARLY WARNINGS

One of the first negative reactions to tobacco came from the Roman Catholic Church in Mexico, which in 1575 passed a law prohibiting smoking in houses of worship. In a German publication, "De plantis epitome utilissima" in 1586, tobacco was labeled a "violent herb." By 1604, King James I of England had increased the import tax on tobacco by 4,000%. In his pamphlet, "A Counterblast to Tobacco," James I called tobacco use "a custome lathsome to the eye, hateful to the nose, harmeful to the braine, dangerous to the lungs, and the blacke stinking fume thereof, nearest resembling the horrible Stigian smoke of the pit that is bottomlesse."

In 1606, King Philip III of Spain declared that tobacco should be grown only in Cuba, Santo Domingo, Venezuela, and Puerto Rico. Sir Francis Bacon, writing in 1610, declared that tobacco use was increasing, and that its use was a habit difficult to stop. In 1612 an imperial edict was issued in China prohibiting the growing or use of tobacco. Dr. William Vaughn warned in his 1617 verse:

Tobacco that outlandish weede
It spends the braine and spoiles the seede
It dulls the spirite, it dims the sight

It robs a woman of her right.

In 1619 the first shipment of women arrived in Jamestown, intended to serve as wives for the new settlers. Their intended husbands were moved to pay for their shipment with 120 pounds of tobacco per wife. That same year, in Berkeley, Virginia, the first American Thanksgiving was celebrated in honor of a bountiful tobacco crop. A year later 40,000 pounds of Virginia tobacco were exported to England.

Then the pendulum swung hard against its use. In 1632, Massachusetts forbade smoking in public. The following year, Sultan Murad IV of Turkey ordered tobacco users executed as infidels. Up to 18 violators a day were put to death. The next year, in Russia, Czar Alexis declared the harshest of penalties for smoking: the first offense was addressed with a whipping, the smoker's nose being split, and exile in Siberia. The penalty for the second offense was death.

The Turkish ban was lifted in 1647, when tobacco joined coffee, wine, and opium as one of the "cushions on the sofa of pleasure." In America, the Colony of Connecticut General Court limited smoking to those at least 21 years of age, unless prescribed to do so by a physician. In 1665, London's famous diarist, Samuel Pepys, wrote of a Royal Society experiment where a cat was given a drop of distilled oil of tobacco—and dropped over dead.

During the 18th century, snuff was king. Sales of other tobacco products, like cigars and cigarettes, were limited to about 10% of the total consumption. In the mid-18th century, a detractor described tobacco as a narcotic akin to opium, and warned that sniffing snuff could result in the loss of the sense of smell, addiction, nasal tumors, and cancer. In England, King George III's wife became known as "Snuffy Charlotte."

Napoleon was rumored to have consumed 7 pounds of snuff per month.

AMERICAN TOBACCO

Tobacco was entwined with the American economy from early on in its history. George Washington, upon marrying Martha Dandridge Custis, added her 286 slaves to his own 30. They were industriously put to work on the 17,000 acres his wife's dowry had brought him, and in 1759 he celebrated the harvesting of his first tobacco crop. The American Revolution that Washington successfully led was partially brought about by the annoying taxes placed by the British on tobacco grown in the Colonies. Yet 5 million pounds of Virginia tobacco served as collateral for the loan Benjamin Franklin secured from France to finance the Revolution.

American Indians, as well as Aztecs and Mayans in Mexico, had been known to use hollow reeds, cane, or maize to craft cigarette-like cylinders stuffed with tobacco. Later, natives of Seville, Spain, fashioned crude cigarettes from discarded paper and cigar scraps. Yet the first modern cigarettes were rolled by an Egyptian artilleryman. In 1832, in the Turk-Egyptian War, he and his crew had discovered that by rolling gunpowder in paper tubes, they were able to increase the rate of their cannon fire. For their performance, they were awarded a pound of tobacco. The only pipe they possessed was broken, so they imitated their gunpowder technique to roll cigarettes from their tobacco store. Their discovery soon spread to both the Egyptian and Turk forces, then eventually around the world.

Tobacco continued being vilified, yet omnipresent. In 1836 the *New England Almanack and Farmers Friend* reported that tobacco was an insecticide, a poison, a filthy habit, and could kill. In the 1855 report of the New York Anti-Tobacco Society, it was labeled a fashionable poison, an addictive substance that caused the deaths of half of those who smoked it between the ages of 35 and 50. Yet that same obnoxious weed was heavily taxed during the U.S. Civil War to help pay for weapons and ammunition. By 1860, manufactured cigarettes had appeared to challenge the dominance of chewing tobacco, snuff, pipe tobacco, and cigars. And from 1861-1865, tobacco was distributed as part of the rations given to soldiers from both the North and South.

LUNG CANCER

In 1889 there were only 140 documented cases of lung cancer reported worldwide. It was not until 1912 that Dr. I. Adler reported that there was strong evidence suggesting a link between lung cancer and smoking. Just two years later, the death rate from lung cancer was 0.6 per 100,000 population, with 371 cases reported in the United States alone. During World War I, American troops were issued cigarettes in their rations, addicting an entire generation to tobacco. General John J. Pershing observed, "You ask me what we need to win this war. I answer, tobacco as much as bullets."

In 1919 Alton Ochsner, a medical student, was invited to observe a surgery for lung cancer. He was told this was an opportunity to witness a procedure he might never again witness in his lifetime. Indeed, for 17 years, he was to see no such surgery again. Yet in the 6 months following that hiatus, he witnessed 8 such operations—every one of them an ex-soldier from World War I who had become hooked on nicotine during the war. By 1925 the rate of lung cancer death had soared to 1.7 per 100,000 population. In 1930 it was 3.8 per

100,000 with 2,357 deaths. During World War II, President Roosevelt proclaimed tobacco a protected crop, and soldiers were once again issued cigarettes in their C-rations. 7,121 cases of lung cancer were reported in the United States in 1940. By that time Americans were smoking an average of over 7 cigarettes per day per adult.

In 1950 Doll and Hill reported in the *British Medical Journal* that heavy smokers were 50 times more likely to develop lung cancer than nonsmokers. In the United States, Wynder and Graham discovered that over 96% of lung cancer patients were moderate-to-heavy chain smokers. By 1956 the lung cancer death rate among white males had risen to 31.0 per 100,000. 29,000 people would die that year alone of lung cancer.

It was not until 1975 that the U.S. military stopped distributing cigarettes as part of their C-rations and K-rations. In 1985, lung cancer surpassed breast cancer as the #1 killer of women in the United States. In 1996, scientists discovered that a benzopyrene derivative, a component of tobacco tar, renders our cancer-suppressor genes ineffective. But it was not until 1999 that Philip Morris, a major tobacco producer and marketer, confessed under pressure that there existed "an overwhelming medical and scientific consensus that cigarette smoking causes lung cancer, heart disease, emphysema and other serious diseases in smokers," and that "cigarette smoking is addictive."

POPULARITY

In 1930 the federal government realized over 50 million dollars from tobacco-use taxes. When the 1934 Garrison Act declared marijuana and other drugs illegal, tobacco was not even mentioned. By 1939, 53% of adult males in the U.S. were smoking, while that figure rose to 66% for those under the age of 40. By 1950, tobacco had invaded television commercials. A frolicking group of cheerleaders were seen chanting the accolades of Lucky Strikes: "Yes, Luckies get our loudest cheers on campus and on dates. With college gals and college guys, a Lucky really rates."

In 1952, Kent cigarettes with the "Micronite" filter were introduced, proclaimed by P. Lorillard's publicity to be "the greatest health protection in history." The filter was made of asbestos. CBS' 1955 "See It Now," hosted by Edward R. Murrow, a chain smoker himself, explored the link between smoking cigarettes and lung cancer, as well as other diseases. Murrow, himself, was to die of lung cancer in 1965.

Dr. Winea J. Simpson, in the 1957 "American Journal of Obstetrics and Gynecology," wrote that the children of smokers tended to be born prematurely, weigh less than normal, and be more susceptible to be stillborn, or die within a month of birth. That same year, U.S. Senator Bennett introduced a bill that would require cigarette packs to carry the warning, "Prolonged use of this product may result in cancer, in lung, heart and circulatory ailments, and in other diseases." Yet by 1964, there were 70 million smokers in the U.S., generating $8 billion for the tobacco industry. The following year, Congress passed a law requiring all cigarette packs to carry the Surgeon General's watered-down warning: "Caution: Cigarette Smoking May Be Hazardous to Your Health." A 1994 Canadian study reported finding traces of cigarette smoke in fetal hair.

PROPAGANDA

In 1972, an internal memorandum from the vice-president of the Tobacco Institute to its president was uncovered. It

134

describes the tobacco industry's strategy of ongoing litigation and manipulation of public opinion to exploit the doubts of the public on the certainty of the claims that tobacco use was harmful, as "brilliantly conceived and executed." It goes on to recommend continued lobbying, and intensified public relations efforts to cast the shadow of doubt on the claim that smoking damages the smoker's health.

In a similar memorandum within RJ Reynolds, a research scientist called the tobacco industry a "specialized, highly ritualized and stylized segment of the pharmaceutical industry." He further declared that, "Tobacco products, uniquely, contain and deliver nicotine, a potent drug with a variety of physiological effects...[and] Happily for the tobacco industry, nicotine is both habituating and unique in its variety of physiological actions, hence no other active material or combination of materials provides equivalent 'satisfaction.'" In the following year, in still another self-incriminating report from RJ Reynolds, a cigarette is defined as "a system for delivery of nicotine to the smoker in attractive, useful form. [The] nicotine occurs in free form, which is rapidly absorbed by the smoker and...instantly perceived as a nicotine kick."

SECOND-HAND SMOKE

In the Surgeon General's report of 1982, second-hand smoke is indicated as a possible cause of lung cancer. This theory was first advocated in 1936 in Germany by Fritz Lickint, who used the term "passive smoking" (*Passivrauchen*). The year following the Surgeon General's report on second-hand smoke, the Surgeon General asserted that smoking was a principal cause of coronary heart disease. By 1987, 44% of all cigarette and cigar smokers had quit. By 1990, smoking was banned on all domestic flights of fewer than 6 hours, with the exception of Alaska and Hawaii. Smoking was also banned on interstate buses. By 1993, smoking amongst U.S. adults had declined to 25% of the population. Yet in that same year, cigarette advertising represented over $6 billion. In Lebanon in 2001, a Shiite Muslim cleric issued a religious edict for his followers to stop smoking. He declared that, "A smoker is committing two crimes, one against himself and the other against the one inhaling next to him."

TARGETING CHILDREN

As far back as 1983, the creative director in a New York advertising agency confessed that they were targeting 14-year-olds to get them to begin smoking. A study done in 1991 revealed that over 90% of 6-year-olds could identify Joe Camel as the symbol for a brand of cigarettes. And from the time Joe Camel was introduced in 1987, up to 1991, the share of Camel cigarettes' under-18 market had risen from 0.5% to 32.8%. Yet a 1992 Gallup survey revealed that 70% of all smokers between the ages of 12 and 17 wished they had never begun smoking. Over half had made a serious attempt to quit, but had failed.

A 1997 study stated that the average age of a first-time smoker was 13, and that more than 3 million adolescents were hooked on cigarettes. The North Texas Medical Group reported in 2001 that 36% of all high school students smoke. Over 15 million children are exposed to secondhand smoke in their homes. Every year 900 million packs of cigarettes are illegally sold to children, with revenues of $1.5 billion. Research indicates that children are more influenced by cigarette advertising than by peer pressure. It can be assumed that 5 million of those under-aged smokers will eventually die a pathetic death from tobacco-related causes.

WARNING LABELS

In 1994 Canadian legislation was proposed to place warning labels on cigarette packs:

"Cigarettes are addictive."
"Tobacco smoke can harm your children."
"Cigarettes cause fatal lung disease."
"Cigarettes cause cancer."
"Smoking during pregnancy can harm your baby."
"Smoking can kill you."
"Tobacco smoke causes fatal lung disease in non-smokers."

BRAIN CHEMISTRY

Nicotine has been shown to increase the neurotransmitter dopamine, which acts on the circuits in the brain that respond with reward and pleasure. By stimulating alpha and beta-adrenergic and dopaminergic receptors, dopamine plays a key role in the regulation of the cardiovascular, renal, hormonal, and central nervous systems. In this sense, nicotine is identical in magnitude and duration to alcohol, amphetamines, cocaine, heroin, and marijuana. It is a highly addictive substance that is both a stimulant and sedative to the central nervous system.

The "kick" the smoker experiences is due to the release of epinephrine from the adrenal cortex, which serves to stimulate the central nervous system as well as other endocrine glands, releasing a burst of glucose. Depression and fatigue soon follow, necessitating another intake of nicotine to sustain the "high." Some 30 seconds after smoke from cigarettes, cigars, or pipes enters the lungs, nicotine floods the brain, remaining in high concentrations for up to 30 minutes.

The beta 3 subunit of the nicotine cholinergic receptor is the critical component in the addiction to nicotine. Some people have a genetic variant that decreases the action of the CYP2A6 enzyme, slowing the decomposition of nicotine, and thus protecting them from nicotine addiction. Normally the stress hormone corticosterone diminishes the impact of nicotine, so more nicotine must be ingested to achieve the same level of intoxication. The net effect of this greater tolerance is increased dependence. Heavy smokers exhibit anger, hostility, aggression, and diminished social cooperation as withdrawal symptoms.

When attempting withdrawal, you must be aware that smoking is a formidable habit that should be gradually diminished to reduce the severity of withdrawal symptoms. During the first few weeks and months of the attempted withdrawal, relapse is common, yet markedly reduced after an abstinence of 3 months. Abstinence is a foreboding challenge, given the constant reminders in advertising, the associations with the practice of smoking, and the inordinate cravings. Techniques such as nicotine gum, the nicotine trans-dermal patch, sprays, and inhalers are effective when combined with behavioral treatment.

THE COSTS

The social and monetary costs of smoking are astronomical. Every day more people succumb to the ills of smoking than die from alcohol, AIDS, car accidents, illegal drugs, murders, and suicides combined. Even secondhand smoke is responsible for over 49 thousand deaths a year.

Health care due to tobacco use is nearly $100 billion annually, while tobacco advertising accounts for $15 billion in the same period. Federal candidates and political parties yearly receive millions of dollars in direct contributions from tobacco companies. Just lobbying Congress during 1998 cost tobacco interests over $58 million. Yet at the same time, it is estimated that work absences, declines in job performance, and early job termination due to tobacco-related health problems cost Americans $40 billion a year. It seems that tobacco and its greed-at-all-costs pushers are a deadly combination of virulent cancers on our society.

TO QUIT

First, *you* must decide to quit. Really. You will experience the craving to smoke from the moment you stop smoking, and that craving will build to a peak in 3-4 days, then gradually lose intensity and frequency. Set a symbolic target date to begin, and then note it down on your calendar. You subsequently can note down your observations, insights, and goals in a diary format. Withdrawal from this deadly drug entails sudden mood changes, frustration, cravings, hunger, fatigue, and difficulty concentrating. Because those seemingly over-powering emotions originate from within you, you must learn to deal with them.

Get rid of all tobacco that might tempt you. Distract yourself when your thoughts stray to smoking. Stand and stretch. Drink a glass of water. Breathe deeply, and remember that you, and only you, are in control of your destiny. Remember why you quit, and say it out loud to yourself. Those gnawing, incessant cravings are a positive sign that you are on your way to getting better. And even intense cravings subside in a few minutes—it does not take a cigarette to make them go away.

Drink a glass of water, chew some gum, or place a piece of candy in your mouth. Celebrate every minute, every day of liberation. Take a walk, and take the time to look around your new world. Keep your hands busy. Talk to someone who can lend support to your efforts. Do not frequent places where people smoke. Do not let your mind ponder places and things that stimulate your desire to smoke. Remember, urges are just urges, nothing more. To be in control, you must tame them. Help yourself by consuming less caffeine, and by keeping away from alcohol. Vary your routine to stimulate your mind. Focus on a healthy diet, knowing that your taste for a whole spectrum of foods will be enhanced every day you stay away from smoke.

Take it a step at a time, a day at a time, and be proud of your progress on your journey. Look stress in the face: write down what causes it, and what approaches you can take to minimize it. You are your own best friend, so act like it. Do not minimize the importance of your struggle—you are undergoing withdrawal symptoms from a highly addictive drug. Be positive. Eat, drink, and exercise healthy. Keep your meals and sleeping on schedule. Listen to soothing music. Close your eyes and meditate on peaceful scenes and pleasant memories. Keep sailing on a steady course, and you can navigate the ocean that seems at first to stretch endlessly to the horizon, yet will soon lie behind you. Do this as if your life depended upon it—it does!

Cigarette smoking and tobacco consumption are pervasive habits that can only be overcome by a passionate will, and by persistently following a plan. You must first understand that you have been the victim (as Buddha would say) of false desires, even though they seem to come from deep within your very being—as true and undeniable as hunger, thirst, sex, sleep, love, ecstasy, or anger. The decisive difference is that those urges to smoke are artificial, not to mention highly detrimental to your physical and spiritual well-being. The sooner you rid yourself of the demon weed of nicotine once and for all, the better off you will be—not to mention all those around you. Make up your mind to cure yourself, and then give it a try.

First, drink a glass of refreshing water, and then follow your own healthy food trail. Exercise a little, but be consistent. Drink heartily from the Fountain of Life, but avoid the poison nicotine as you would the plague. Good luck. We are all with you.

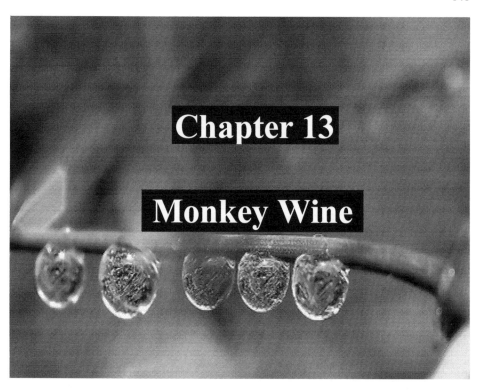

Chapter 13

Monkey Wine

"Upon the first goblet he read this inscription, *monkey wine*; upon the second, *lion wine*; upon the third, *sheep wine*; upon the fourth, *swine wine*. These four inscriptions expressed the four descending degrees of drunkenness: the first, that which enlivens; the second, that which irritates; the third, that which stupefies; finally the last, that which brutalizes."

—Victor Hugo

ETHYL ALCOHOL

Ethyl alcohol is the intoxicating agent in liquor. This organic compound of carbon, hydrogen, and oxygen—CH_3CH_2OH—is produced by the fermentation of sugars and starches. The biological oxidation of carbohydrates occurs when a naturally occurring yeast consumes the sugars and starches in fruits, berries, honey, flowers, milk, and so on, and secretes alcohol as a by-product. Alcohol is naturally found scattered throughout the human body in minute quantities—in the brain, blood, liver, muscles, and in bacteria found in the large intestine. But ethyl alcohol (i.e., ethanol) most commonly finds its way into the human body by drinking.

When consumed, alcohol immediately modifies one's behavior, initially making the drinker feel relaxed and tranquil, reducing the level of anxiety, and increasing the sense of confidence. When more than 6 ounces are consumed, the initial euphoria that is produced is transformed into a depression. Because the liver can only metabolize about one ounce of alcohol per hour, any amount greater than that produces intoxication lasting from 1 to 12 hours. Surveys indicate that over 7% of all Americans, or some 20 million individuals, currently abuse and/or are dependent on alcohol. In our pursuit of health and happiness, alcohol abuse has to be taken into serious account.

ANCIENT HISTORY

Since near the beginning of man's history, he has known of alcohol by way of the spoiled fruit and juices that contain its intoxicating spirit. Simple foods like honey, dates, and even sap, if left alone to ferment, produce alcohol. Early on in his history, man's body evolved the enzyme *alcohol dehydrogenase* to detoxify himself. (Half of the population in Asia lack this enzyme, making it uncomfortable for them to ingest alcohol.) Archeological evidence indicates that wine was being produced in Mesopotamia (i.e., modern Iraq and eastern Syria) at least 5,000 years ago. Recipes for more than 20 varieties of beer were recorded on clay tablets. At the same time, extensive crops of wheat and barley were produced in the fertile river deltas of Egypt and Mesopotamia to serve as cereal diets for a growing population.

It did not take long for these ancients to discover and proliferate the consumption of barley and wheat beers. Also at about the same time, Chinese and Egyptians left written evidence of vineyards and wine production. Egyptian frescos reveal festive grape harvests, with the finest blends of the ensuing wine meant for the pharaohs. A Sumerian cuneiform tablet dated to 2100 B.C. is a pharmacopoeia of recipes, amongst which are descriptions of alcohol use. Hippocrates prescribed wine for a wide variety of acute and chronic ailments. Even taxes could be paid with wine.

Around 2,000 B.C., the code of Babylonian king Hammurabi proscribed the approved method of buying and selling wine, and the punishments to be dealt out to those who violated the code. By 800 B.C., barley and rice wine were being distilled in India. Around 50 B.C., Dionysius of Halicarnassus noted that, "the Gauls (i.e., French) have no knowledge of wine, but used a foul-smelling liquor made of barley rotted in water." The ancient Greeks shipped their wine abroad in storage vessels coated with resin to prevent leakage. The resin lent a turpentine taste to their wine. To alter the taste before consumption, the wine was flavored with spices, herbs, flowers, or perfumes, and then heavily diluted with water.

The Roman god of wine, Bacchus, oversaw the planting and harvesting of grapes, as well as the ceremonies and festivities associated with wine. Roman vineyards extended from modern-day Italy to Greece, Spain, France, and Germany. Extensive production and trade occurred in and around the Mediterranean from the very beginnings of commerce. When the Roman dominance of Europe came unraveled in the 5th century A.D., the Catholic Church carried on its viniculture.

The far-flung monastic orders produced wine not only for sacramental use, but also as a source of revenue. They experimented with the forerunners of brandies and other liqueurs based on wine. By 1100, alcohol distillation was being practiced in the medical school at Salerno, Italy. They aptly named the concentrated alcohol "spirits," being the mere essence of wine. By the 17th century, alcohol, along with hashish and opium, had become popular in Constantinople (today Istanbul, Turkey).

A HEALTHY DRINK

Early on, the increasingly sophisticated use of agricultural techniques led to food surpluses, which resulted in greater populations living in close quarters. While the majority of water supplies were contaminated and unhealthy to the general population, alcoholic beverages proved to be a safe source of fluids and calories. Most fruit juices are too naturally low in sugar content to ferment sufficiently, but with the advent of agriculture, selected varieties were cultivated with a higher sugar content that allowed for easier fermentation. Even the Old and New Testaments of the *Bible* make few references to water as the beverage of choice.

Some of the few references made by the ancient Greeks are those of Hippocrates who wrote of the refreshing waters borne of mountain springs, and of wells and collected rainwater. In the Middle Ages, alcohol, this most popular and common drink was labeled *aqua vitae*, the water of life. In the colorful fairs held in French and Flemish towns, wine took center stage. Great quantities were purchased in the Bordeaux region by the British to be exported to England. Yet we should be reminded that diluted alcoholic beverages were consumed more to quench thirst and nourish than for intoxication. They were an abundant source of micronutrients that added needed vitamins and minerals to the diet. Beyond nutrition, the boredom and weariness of daily life was assuaged by diluted wines and beers. It has only been in the last century that the masses have had easy access to an abundant supply of safe drinking water, and potent alcohols intended to stupefy and seduce the senses.

Man's relationship to alcohol has recently changed. Historically, alcoholic drinks reduced harmful bacteria to permit drinking otherwise unhealthy water. It hydrated, fed, and maintained the equilibrium of entire populations. It was used ceremonially to honor marriages, births, and deaths. Friends were welcomed and taken leave of by warm toasts to their health and happiness. New events were celebrated by drink—new projects, achievements, new years, and harvests. Ships were launched, journeys begun, victories celebrated, and defeats commiserated. The wealthy celebrated their good fortunes, and the poor attempted to drown out a few moments of the agony of their poverty. Alcohol has been an elixir to society for millennia.

EARLY PROHIBITION

Shortly before 100 A.D., the Roman Emperor Domitian, concerned that the populace was drinking too heavily, ordered half the vineyards destroyed, and curtailed the planting of new vineyards. His movement spread to other countries, but without success. His prohibition was soon repealed. In fact, most early laws were aimed at the consequences brought on by excessive drinking, not at the drinking in and of itself. Hebrew laws considered infractions of the law with equal punishment, whether the perpetrator was drunk or sober. Yet Roman law tended to punish the inebriated perpetrator less severely than the sober one. The early Church did not consider drinking a sin. Castigation was reserved for drunkenness, especially for the offending clergy. During the Middle Ages, as the Church's influence spread, its dictates became incorporated into common law. The Far and Near Eastern religions forbade drinking as a violation of natural law emanating from the corrupted Christian world. The vehement condemnation of abusive drinking by the Christian Church as sinful and immoral did not emerge until the 17th and 18th centuries with the Protestant Reformation. Calvin and Luther preached temperance, blaming the breakdown of family life, licentiousness, and public inebriety on the seduction of alcohol.

DISTILLATION

Distillation was promoted in England in the 18th century. Due to the animosity that persisted between the English and the French, the immense quantities of light wines that flowed into England from France were taxed with stiff tariffs, with the intention that the heavy wines of Portugal would replace them. Dutch gin (a product of fermented, then distilled cereal grains) was smuggled into the country until the British began wholesale distillation of English gin. To produce their gin, the British began by distilling pure spirits, and then redistilling them with juniper berries and small amounts of diverse ingredients like anise seed, cardamom seed, coriander seed, orange peel, cassia bark, and fennel. The end product was not aged.

Almost overnight, England converted from a beer-and-ale (8% alcoholic content), and port-wine (18-22% alcoholic content) society, to a hard-liquor, gin (35-45% alcoholic content) society. This stupefying liquor was cheap, easily accessible, and highly promoted. By the middle of the 18th century, the policy shifted to one of discouraging gin consumption with increasingly higher taxes, the licensing of pubs, and restrictive regulations on the manner, terms, and times that alcohol could be sold. These laws forced the society to turn away from hard liquors to the former consumption of beers and ales.

America also rode the wave of distilled liquors. Although the original colonists had subsisted on home-brewed beer, ale, and wine, they began importing rum (fermented, then distilled sugar-cane juice) from the Caribbean in the 1600s, and then soon began distilling their own gin and whisky. The churches in the Colonies established drunkenness as a sin, and converted that credence into secular law. The original Puritan penchant for fines, flogging, imprisonment, and censure have persevered up to the time of our contemporary society.

A plethora of early laws focused on the manufacture, sale, and trafficking of intoxicating beverages. Innkeepers were discouraged from permitting gambling and drunkenness, yet the true intent of colonial lawmakers was not to somehow modify the causes nor the effects of abusive drinking, but rather to benefit personally from the economic and political ramifications of the industry.

By the last half of the 18th century, whisky was being distilled from fermented grain mashes throughout the United States. Bourbon whisky was produced to avoid high grain taxes and reduce corn and grain crops in bulk for easier transportation and distribution. Whisky became America's new medium of exchange. In the 1820s and 1830s, religious revivalism focused on temperance and the abolition of slavery. The first prohibition law was passed in Maine, in 1846. Leaders in the prohibition movement feared the effects of the rampant growth of the cities (where most debauchery took place).

Simultaneously, the evangelical Protestant middle classes were becoming increasingly anti-alien and anti-Roman Catholic.

SALOONS AND PROHIBITION

With the waves of Scandinavian and German immigrants after the American Civil War, came a traditional preference for beer that gradually changed America's drinking habits. By 1890, beer had surpassed hard liquor as America's favorite alcoholic drink. Radical technological advances in railroads, the telegraph, and mechanical refrigeration amongst others, had made possible the birth of vertically integrated companies in the beer business.

Pabst Brewing Company of Milwaukee, Wisconsin, and Annheuser Busch of St. Louis, Missouri, were aggressive producers and marketers of their beers. To penetrate new markets, they supplied the capital to establish their own saloons. There was suddenly a massive expansion of saloons, many towns having one for every 200 inhabitants. With greater competition came more competitive marketing: free lunches were offered, as well as gambling, cock-fighting, and prostitution. These dens of depravity were an eyesore to many members of the community.

In 1893 the Anti-Saloon League was formed to politicize the reform movement. They were joined in battle by the Woman's Christian Temperance Union and other dry organizations to prohibit the importing, exporting, transporting, selling, and manufacturing of intoxicating liquor. Their success was manifested in the Eighteenth Amendment to the United States Constitution, which took effect on January 29, 1920. Even before that time, prohibition was already law in 33 states, affecting nearly two-thirds of the population. On October 28, 1919, the National Prohibition Act, better known as the

Volstead Act, was passed, declaring alcohol consumption illegal. The minimum content of intoxicating liquor was defined as 0.5%, and guidelines were created for enforcement, as well as exemption of alcohol for use in medicine and sacraments.

Alcohol consumption was soon reduced to 30% of its former levels, and there was reason to believe the prohibitionists' goals were actually obtainable: improved health and hygiene; reduced crime, poverty, and death rates; and an improved economy. Unfortunately, this proved not to be the case. Prohibition was unenforceable—it led to a notable increase in crime, and actually resulted in an increased consumption of alcoholic beverages. Murders increased by over 75%. Al Capone's Chicago was the stage for over 400 gangland murders a year.

In 1927, Capone's organization comprised of hundreds of employees and thousands of outlets, grossed $60 million from alcohol, and $25 million from gambling. Bootleggers flagrantly violated the law, smuggling quantities of liquor from Canada and abroad, manufacturing their own, and even stealing it from government warehouses. Only 5% of the illicit flow of liquor was curtailed by authorities, who, more often than not, were accomplices. Speakeasies replaced saloons. By 1925 there were over 100,000 speakeasies in New York City alone. It is now generally agreed that organized crime mushroomed during prohibition. Legal jobs decreased, law enforcement suffered both in image and effectiveness, violence thrived, and black-market prices for alcohol escalated.

Because beer proved to be too bulky to be profitable, hard liquor came into vogue. It seemed that nearly everywhere; wholesale quantities of bathtub gin were being fortified by additives and chemicals of all sorts. By 1925, over 4,000 people a year were dying from poisoned liquor. Arrests for drunk driving increased by over 80%, and arrests for drunkenness and disorderly conduct went up by over 40%. There was a proliferation of home products that could be fermented to produce wine and beer. The sale of medicinal alcohol—95% pure—increased by 400%. For many riding the heady tide of the Roaring Twenties, alcohol became the symbol of their personal freedom of self-expression and hedonistic pleasure. For the Drys, often rural and small-town fundamentalists, Prohibition was a noble, yet flawed experiment, doomed to failure from the onset.

For the Wets, most commonly city dwellers, it simply glorified their rebellious assertion that they had the innate right to intoxication. Nearly everyone became disenchanted with the criminal involvement in the production and sale of liquor, the explosive popularity of the speakeasies, and the increased restriction of personal liberties. The Prohibition Amendment, the 18th, was repealed by the 21st Amendment, ratified on December 5, 1933, just 9 months after the new Democratic President, Franklin D. Roosevelt, took office. A few states continued prohibiting the consumption of alcohol, and it was not until 1966 that all had given up in futility.

FETAL ALCOHOL SYNDROME

Fetal Alcohol Syndrome, first recognized as such in 1968, has become the leading identified cause of mental retardation in the world. Pregnant women who are consistently heavy drinkers, or even those who engage in occasional binge drinking, are responsible for over 5,000 defective births every year in the United States alone. Approximately 40% of the women who consume large quantities of alcohol during their pregnancies will give birth to a child with Fetal Alcohol

Syndrome, while about 10% of moderate drinkers risk the same sad outcome. Congenital defects are most commonly a result of drinking during the first trimester, and premature birth and low birth weight are results of drinking during the last trimester.

Of those 3 babies in 1,000 who are born to drinking mothers, the average I.Q. of the child is 63. They also suffer from motor retardation, inferior muscle tone, and hearing problems. Many have facial deformities: small eyes with short eye openings, an underdeveloped upper lip, and flattening of the upper lip ridges. They are likely to suffer from a heart murmur for their first year of life, and can be haunted by heart irregularities like ventricular or atrial septal defect the rest of their lives.

These babies are born small, and develop slowly. Bonding with their mothers may be difficult. They may exhibit delays in walking, overall coordination, language assimilation, and toilet training. They begin as irritable babies, who soon grow into hyperactive children with attention deficits. These children of alcohol often exhibit antisocial behaviors: lying, stealing, defiance of authority, sexual promiscuity, and violence. One study of a group of 18-year-olds with Fetal Alcohol Syndrome, revealed their academic level to be equivalent to that of 4th graders. What a sad inheritance to pass on to one's own child.

TREATMENT

Nearly 19 million Americans suffer from alcohol abuse. Over 3.5 million are dependent on drugs like marijuana, cocaine, and pain relievers. Nearly 72 million are hooked on tobacco products. Up to 90% of all Americans commonly ingest caffeine in their sodas and coffee—the most-used mood-altering drug in the world. 4 million U.S. adults are addicted to food. Gambling seriously affects up to 8 million adults. 20%

of the adult population is addicted to shopping. 16 million are addicted to compulsive sexual behavior. Even the Internet is considered to be an impulse-control disorder of gigantic proportions. Yet, where there is a will, there is a way out.

Rats and monkeys, who are not particularly renown for their willpower, are commonly used as subjects of laboratory experiments. In such a setting, they have been observed voluntarily consuming large amounts of cocaine, opioids, and alcohol. They, like their drug-dependent human counterparts, spend inordinate amounts of time and energy locating, consuming, yet ultimately recovering from their drug habits.

Both people, as well as addicted lab animals, lose their previous focus on family, friends, recreation and work in order to pursue the demands placed on them by their drug habits. It has been noted in lab experiments that drug use is promoted by stress, fear, nervousness, threat, social isolation, lack of food and drink, and exercise. As the deliberative cognition of the prefrontal cortex is subverted, addicts become more impulsive.

Every day more than 700,000 people in the United States receive treatment to control their alcohol addiction. Of those hundreds of thousands, over 13% receive their treatment in an inpatient setting, while the other 86% receive outpatient treatment. Unfortunately, the recovery success rate is only around 20%. Rehabilitation is approximately a 90-day struggle. The first decision is whether the goal is to be that of abstinence or moderation. The choice of goals depends on the drinking history, their physical and psychological dependence on alcohol, and medical considerations.

COGNITIVE-BEHAVIORAL THERAPY

Cognitive-Behavioral Therapy is a non-pharmacological approach aimed at enabling the drinker to identify high-risk situations where relapse is probable, and to develop strategies to recognize and confront the accompanying cravings. The drinker should establish his goals, and be constantly monitoring them and assessing his performance. He should note in his diary the amount of drinks he has allowed himself, and the amount taken in a given time period. He should note the duration of his drinking, where it took place, his companions, any other factors he deems pertinent, and the immediate and long-term outcomes of his drinking.

He should attempt to avoid drinking (or severely reduce it) in times of high stress—when in the company of certain people who stimulate his desire to drink, when he feels anger or frustration, or when other obligations demand his attention. He should develop strategies for refusing a drink, substituting diluted or non-alcoholic drinks, pacing himself by drinking less frequently, or delaying before drinking. He should prepare himself for various settings and situations, motivating himself to self-control, rewarding himself for following his pre-established strategy, and receiving feedback by talking to himself and others as he maneuvers through difficult situations.

THE ALCOHOLICS ANONYMOUS
12-STEP FACILITATION THERAPY

The 12 steps of the Alcoholics Anonymous (AA) recovery process are widely known and have been widely adopted. They are based on the premise that the problem drinker must recognize that by himself, he is incapable of controlling his alcohol consumption. He must make a moral inventory of himself, his habit, and its effects both on himself, as well as those near to him. He must then make a confession of his transgressions. These steps are often combined with therapy, as the drinker conscientiously reads the AA literature, attends AA meetings, obtains a mentor, and keeps a diary of his attendance, participation, and progress.

The angry, indignant, self-pitying drinker is likened to an actor who tries to micromanage his entire life performance. His selfish attempt at playing God is doomed to failure. He must renounce his erroneous strategy, beginning with a heart-felt personal inventory. Those damaged or worthless elements he discovers must be discarded. His growing faith gives him courage to overcome his own insecurities. As he successfully moves through these 12 steps, he gradually takes control of his own life, and becomes whole. To successfully achieve his transition, he must:

1. Admit he was powerless over alcohol, and that his life had become unmanageable.

2. Come to believe that a Power greater than himself could restore him to sanity.

3. Make a decision to turn his will and his life over to the care of God (as he understands Him).

4. Make a searching and fearless moral inventory of himself.

5. Confess to God, to himself, and to another human being the exact nature of his wrongs.

6. Be entirely ready to have God remove all his defects of character.

7. Humbly ask God to remove his shortcomings.

8. Make a list of all persons he has harmed, and become willing to make amends to them all.

9. Make direct amends, whenever possible, to the persons he has harmed, except when to do so would injure them or others.

10. Continue to take personal inventory, and promptly admit when he is wrong.

11. Seek through prayer and meditation to improve his conscious contact with God (as he understands Him), praying only for knowledge of His will, and the power to carry out that will.

12. Experience a spiritual awakening as the result of these steps, try to carry this message to other alcoholics, and practice these principles in all his affairs.

PHARMACOTHERAPY

The two types of medical treatments practiced by therapists involve aversive medications and anti-craving medications. The most popular of the aversive medications is *disulfiram*, which is intended to create havoc with the drinker when he ingests alcohol. His heart begins to race, his blood pressure soars, he feels flush, nauseous, and begins to vomit. Disulfiram has been in use for over 50 years, yet the results of this treatment are mixed.

Naltrexone is the preferred anti-craving medication. Its intent is to reduce the pleasant effects of alcohol and the subsequent cravings by interfering with the brain's endogenous opioids that result in the euphoria and loss of anxiety triggered by alcohol. Like disulfiram, treatment with naltrexone has been practiced for some 50 years. It was originally reported to reduce relapses after a period of 3 months from 50% to 25%. These and other treatments are not to be taken lightly. They result from consultation and evaluation from an alcoholism treatment specialist, or a primary care provider.

You must realize that unhealthy habits can be replaced by healthy habits. Just give it a try.

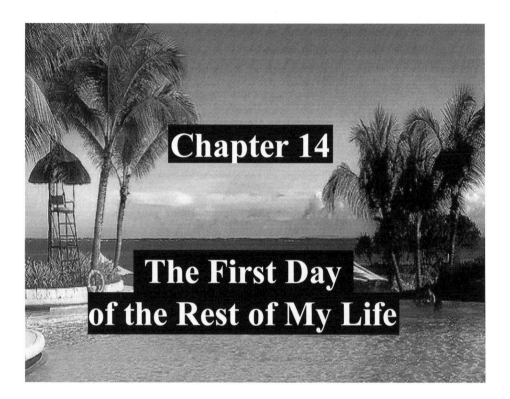

Chapter 14

The First Day
of the Rest of My Life

PAUL'S STORY

I am a creature of habit. My routine has brought me security, and a comforting regularity in my life. I tend to rise at 6:30 A.M., with or without my alarm clock. I seem to carry around an internal buzzer that snaps me out of sleep as soon as the sun rises. This is not something I have willed, or perfected from long practice, but just something innate, a real part of me that I never really question. Once awake, there is no need to take stock of what awaits me, nor the water I have tread the previous day. I simply roll out of bed, throw on a nightshirt, and head for the kitchen. My cat meows as I pass his bed. My children stir in their beds, still a dream away from awakening. I pour a cup of milk into a cup, insert it into the microwave oven, then wait 1 minute and 35 seconds for it to heat up, remove it, add two teaspoons of sugar and one of instant Nescafé, stir, take a sip, then set it on the dining room table. In all this, hardly a conscious thought has passed through my mind.

The computer switch is flicked on, and as it warms up, the living room light is also turned on. I peruse my daily calendar to get a sense of the direction my day will take. Call the school to see about tickets to the game this weekend, make sure the phone bill gets paid with a check and sent out today, and remind myself not forget to do the laundry tonight. Mundane, but necessary. So is my breakfast. In fact, this morning I am not in the mood to force down a bowl of cereal, much less a plate of eggs and toast.

It seems that again that initial cup of coffee will have to do me all morning. My stomach is all right with that, until about 10:00 o'clock when it starts to protest. I try to ignore it as if it were some alien urge attempting to interrupt the flow of my routine. Another cup of coffee usually quiets it, yet soon ties my stomach into knots. Oh well, lunch will soon quiet its protests, and get me through the afternoon.

When I snap back to reality, I have already stripped down, showered, shampooed, and shaved, dried off, applied hair cream and deodorant, and wandered back into the bedroom. Now that I am semi-conscious, I deftly pick out pants, shirt, and socks that are themes on the same color. The only true expression of my outlook on the day—determined by the collage of people I expect to see, the tasks that await me, the game face I must wear—is expressed in my tie. Look carefully at my tie, and you will see what I expect from my world and myself at that moment in time. A few practiced flips and it is in place. Shoes, brief case, set the computer for voice mail. Perhaps a goodbye to my wife, who has also begun her daily routine in a haze. Ask me an hour later what I did this morning, and I can tell you nothing. The wonderful thing about a routine is that it is invisible to the consciousness, a truly automatic process per-formed robotically.

CONTENDING WITH COFFEE

Since the day that I began to become aware of my routine and apply some common sense to it, nothing has changed much. I still wake up with or without my alarm clock, still shower and dress automatically, but when I arrive at the kitchen, instead of preparing my coffee, I pour myself a glass of orange juice, take a sip, then continue with my routine. I listen to my stomach when it lets me know it has fasted throughout the night and now wants some sustenance. Now I listen to myself. If I am up to it, I peel and slice an apple or an orange, then savor the slices one by one. That takes the edge off my hunger.

It just takes a minute to prepare a couple of fried eggs (in a dash of olive oil), scrambled eggs, or an omelet. I still follow my routine unconsciously, but I have begun to substitute healthy foods for harmful and useless ones. And if I do still desire that cup of coffee to chip away at that fog of sleep that lingers in my head, I follow it with a glass of water to dilute its aggressive nature.

My stomach is content, and I know that half way through the morning I will not fall into that tailspin that seems to cry out for coffee to stimulate me back up to normal. I have broken the chain of false dependence. My life with coffee has become one of a controlled relationship, and I can feel the difference. Often good dieting comes down to making the right decision, steering the correct course, then setting yourself on autopilot.

160

In the old days, my adrenaline would fire up on my way to work. The traffic seemed like a barrage of buzzing soldier bees bent on stressing me out. I was pushing, competing, always in a hurry, yet never really saving a second of travel time. In a calmer frame of mind, I analyzed those agonizing minutes I spent commuting daily, and realized I could reformat my approach. I began leaving 5 minutes earlier, driving like a sane person for a change—not tail gaiting nor challenging—and began to enjoy the scenery, the music from my radio, the humming flow of the traffic.

The colors of the world are so often painted from within. That whole cloud of stress had been painting my world in grays for far too long. Now when I feel the urge, I reach down beside my car seat and lift up my bottle of water in a toast to my new life. By the time I get to work, I will have drunk the entire bottle, and arrive with a whole new point of view of myself and the colorful world around me.

Without coffee, I feel less artificially awake, and actually more alert and comfortably within my own boundaries. When the 10:00 o'clock urge to eat arrives, the one that used to be drowned in a river of coffee, I pull out a plastic bag with a snack of carrots and celery, and chase it down with a bubbly drink of bottled water. All of this happens automatically, unconsciously, as do all routines. Yet this routine has been carefully thought through, and a solid strategy plotted out. I have set a new course for my life, and not only do I feel more in control than ever, but I can see the results in the faces of others I deal with, in the mirror, and in my own mind's eye.

CONTENDING WITH NICOTINE

Now, coffee was not the only drug I had to deal with. I

smoked like a chimney. A good part of my subconscious motivation to haul myself out of bed in the morning was to saturate my lungs with nicotine. My body and mind were awash with this poison. As a young man, I had imitated not only my friends, but also that sociable, successful man I had often seen in advertisements, puffing away pleasurably, a smiling girl at each arm.

Once I had fallen into the trap, my desire to continue drugging myself was greater than the willpower I needed to climb the slippery walls out of addiction. Everyone else smoked. I could quit whenever I wished. Didn't I deserve a little pleasure in my life? Both my aunts smoked heavily, then suddenly died in agony. Confronting that reality, I began to gain a sense of my own mortality.

The facts that began to emerge confronted me with another possibility: what if this seemingly frivolous enjoyment were really an instrument of death? Was I prepared for the drawn-out torment of lung cancer, the horror of heart disease, the rancid decaying of my body before my own eyes?

As I began to think of a way out, I knew before any strategy could be put into place, that it must be laid on the cornerstone of my own true desire to quit. I began by taking a self-assessment: my breath was putrid, my fingernails yellowed …even my eyes were a glossy yellow. I trembled if I ran out of cigarettes. Like a heroin addict, I constantly needed a fix. My life degenerated to a sick worshiping of the nicotine idol. It was worlds apart from what I had envisioned it to be as a youth—an innocent vehicle to pleasure. It really seemed as if I had boarded a vehicle bound for hell. How was I to get off?

I began by confronting the monster. I read and mulled over articles of science, opinion, and propaganda. I thought.

Once prepared for battle, I quit cold turkey. Yet it was a devious battle, fought on the battleground of my own mind, my own self somehow turned against myself. These cravings were real, and deeply ingrained in my psyche. Yet there was light at the end of the tunnel. I sublimated: when I was dying for a cigarette, I forced myself to think of other things, I got busy, kept myself distracted, and pushed on with my life. I talked to myself, muttering the goals I had set, the promises I had made, with the determination of arriving at my destination.

I drank a glass of water, chewed gum, and my agony converted to the painful pleasure of conquest. But my devious guest came back again and again, always with the promise of relief and respite from this torture. Fortunately, my stubborn faith in a better future, and my own ability to create that future, overcame the beast in me. After the first month, the cravings subsided. But they will be there for a long time, waiting only for an image of smoke, a familiar place, a familiar smell to trigger that devilish desire.

Now when I drive to work, I am not permeating my clothing, to say nothing of my brain, with that obnoxious-smelling smoke. The taste of food has begun to blossom again; my appetite has been reborn. I was worried about gaining weight after quitting smoking, but I discovered that a 15-minute walk in the evening more than offsets the calories that used to go up in smoke. Besides, I would never, never trade this new self for the old, pathetically devalued, stressed-out self I had become.

Now, instead of unconsciously reaching down for another cigarette, another poisoned stick of doom, I reach for my bottle of water and, surprisingly, am subtly stimulated and satisfied to an extent my cigarette could never offer. On the map of human endeavor, in the scope of great accomplishments, mine may seem miniscule, but it is mine, and I treasure it, and thank the Heavens that I woke up and found the strength within myself to set myself on a new course.

I am not distracted by my drug habit any more. I do not smell bad, and am not afraid to get within breathing distance of my coworkers. Instead of focusing on finishing a task in order to take a cigarette break, I focus on the task itself. My heightened pride in my work has brought me greater rewards at work, not to mention the self-satisfaction that comes from a job well done. Now that I have my life better arranged, I want to concentrate on my own and my family's happiness. And it is much easier to see that happiness when you are not straining your eyes through the fog of drugs.

CONTENDING WITH ALCOHOL

Did I mention liquor? Yes, I had a long love affair with booze. There is no doubt that with the anxiety and stress that are inherent in just going through the motions of commuting, meeting deadlines, answering e-mail, calling clients, and dealing with the expectations and demands of bosses, coworkers, and family, a little relief is necessary. I seemed to need a lot of relief. That drink or two after work, became seven or eight, gradually becoming the problem itself instead of the solution.

My mood changed. I could hardly believe the way I growled and barked. Daily I became stoned, staring at the TV in a state of stupefaction, ignoring the richness and texture of the family dynamics going on around me. I was oblivious, supposedly healing my own self-inflicted wounds. No wonder I sensed myself growing indifferent to my family. Why couldn't they reach out to me, allay my suffering, understand my anguish? I guess it's just is not that way.

It took some good, hard counseling from my wife, repeated harsh words and looks from my children, and a good look at myself in the mirror to see my own selfishness and self-indulgence. But once I became aware of the gulf between how I had always envisioned myself, and the person I had become, I was frightened enough to pursue sobriety with enthusiasm.

I finally decided to quit. I knew that there was no going halfway. Later, if I felt so inclined, I would allow myself that drink or two to calm the nerves after a long day, but I could never travel the road to alcoholism again. Never. Every time I felt the urge to take a drink of liquor, I drank a glass of water instead. I consciously concentrated on drinking H_2O, remembering that water is the essence of all life-giving fluids. I served it in a wine glass, admired its clarity, its effervescence, savored it as I drank, and appreciated its life-saving nature.

It worked miracles. After a few days of soaring blood pressure (which I monitored at home, but should have done under my doctor's care), occasional dizziness, fatigue, headaches, and disorientation, I came surging back to reality. I became a new person. I simultaneously pursued a sound diet, which previously had been easily ignored by substituting liquor for food.

SEEKING THE GOOD DIET

Once I had opened my eyes to the possibilities of a good diet, I found endless sources at my fingertips. Dozens of popular magazines carry detailed tips for appetizing foods and simple recipes. New insights and scientific studies are easily accessed on the Internet and at the local library. All it takes is interest, and a little effort. I could not believe that all this information had all along been lying silently at my feet. All I had to do was pick it up and read. I went shopping for fruits and vegetables. Every day we would cut up fresh fruits and vegetables and place them under our noses on the table.

It is amazing how delightful fresh broccoli, cauliflower, carrots, oranges, plums, pears, and kiwi can be. Eating a decent breakfast was another key element. Getting rid of junk food, and simply not bringing it home, eliminated the temptation to snack, or at least diverted it to healthier foods. We began by taking a few extra seconds to prepare well-rounded meals with selected portions of carbohydrates in the form of rice and potatoes. Fruits and vegetables became a staple at every meal. We became more creative in cooking fish and chicken.

Within a week of stopping to drown myself in liquor, and instead, focusing on a sound diet with sufficient water, I emerged a new person. My attention span gradually increased, as did my perception of myself and my surroundings. I began to relate to my family and my coworkers on a different level. It was like awakening from a long dream—not especially from a coma, but more like from a haze that had miraculously lifted from my brain. I was a new person, even when performing mundane tasks like tying my shoes or combing my hair. There was a new sense of vitality, of purpose that had wilted under the abuse of drugs like alcohol and cigarettes.

RECLAIMING MY LIFE

With this new awakening came higher levels of energy. Once my mind had been reclaimed, I suddenly felt like reclaiming my body. I began by making a habit of taking short walks around the neighborhood. Old memories of sights, sounds, and odors swept through me. It was as if I were sensing the world again after a long hiatus. It gave me goose bumps. I had regained a big chunk of my life.

When I finally felt up to begin jogging, I understood the interplay amongst good diet, water, exercise, and no drugs. Instead of helplessly watching myself decline physically and spiritually, I felt myself inch upward as I followed the path of common sense. I have recently begun lifting modest amounts of weights, and feel the reassuring soreness of muscles waking up after a long rest. I will have quite a story to tell my grandchildren.

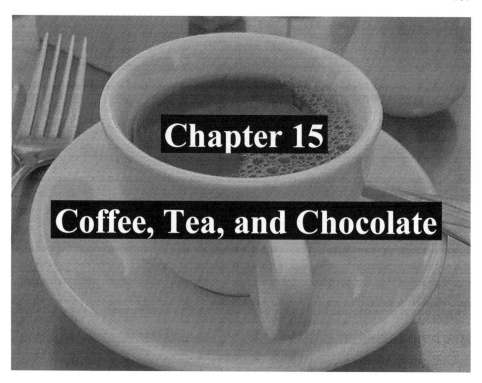

Chapter 15

Coffee, Tea, and Chocolate

THE NATURE OF COFFEE

About 80% of the world's coffee is produced from a shrub or small tree of the genus *Coffea arabica*, which is represented by some 15 varieties. It is found most typically in Brazil, Columbia, Venezuela, Peru, Haiti, Santo Domingo, Guatemala, and El Salvador. Coffee is a tropical plant that requires a moderately cool climate that is moist, but not wet. The coffee tree flowers in profuse clusters of white blossoms that give off a sweet, jasmine-like scent. Its small, pulpy fruit, called a cherry, contains twin seeds, the bluish-green coffee beans, coupled together on the flat surfaces. Each bean is coated with a thin, silvery film, which in turn is enclosed in a type of golden-yellow parchment. Each tree can be expected to yield between 1 to 4 pounds of beans. Once picked by hand, knocked off by poles, or removed by machinery, the fruit can be processed using the Wet Method, or the Dry Method. The former involves pulping and fermenting the berries, allowing them to ferment so the membranes can be easily removed. In the Dry Method, the berries are placed in the sun to dry off before the exocarp is removed by milling.

The extracted green beans are transported to a roasting plant where they are blended with other varieties for flavor, then heated for 5-12 minutes at temperatures varying from 380-1000 degrees Fahrenheit, depending on the desired outcome. Ground and vacuum-packed, the coffee can remain fresh up to 2 years. About one-fifth of all green beans are used in the production of instant coffee, some 40% of those being freeze-dried. The coffee extract for instant coffee is obtained by passing water at a temperature of 350 degrees Fahrenheit through coarsely ground coffee. The liquid is filtered, the water evaporated, then spray-dried. The particles can be agglomerated with steam to form granules, or frozen, freeze-dried in a vacuum for sublimation of the ice crystals. Before packaging, aromas are normally added in a carbon-dioxide or nitrogen atmosphere. Decaffeinated coffee is prepared from green beans softened by steam, then extracted with boiling chlorinated solvents to remove the caffeine. The residual solvent is removed by a second steaming, and then the beans are dried and processed as normal beans.

CAFFEINE

Caffeine is an extremely bitter, crystalline alkaloid, $C_8H_{10}N_4O_2$ (known medically as trimethylxanthine), comprising about 2% of the dry weight of *Coffea Arabica*, as well as significant amounts in tea, cacao, and so on. *Coffea Robusta*, a variety that grows principally in Africa, Asia, and Indonesia, can contain twice the caffeine of its cousin, *Arabica*. Caffeine extends the stimulating effects of AMP (i.e., adenosine mono-phosphate—the principal regulator of the cells' biochemical activity), affecting principally the heart and the central nervous system. It is also a diuretic, causing dehydration by stimulating urination.

COFFEE'S EARLY HISTORY

The discovery of coffee is lost in the shrouds of legend. It is said that somewhat before 850 A.D., an Ethiopian goat herder from Kaffa, named Kaldi, noticed his animals chewing on the red berries of a common shrub. They soon became abnormally active, even restless, and seemed not to tire all night. He tried some of the berries himself, with the same outcome. Soon his discovery had spread, and berries were commonly being wrapped in animal fat, coming into popular use as a stimulant. By 1100, the first coffee bushes were being cultivated in Turkey, Yemen, Arabia, and Egypt, yielding beans that were roasted and boiled much as we do today. The Turks added anise, cardamom, cinnamon, and clove to flavor the bitter brew which they called *qahwa* (i.e., that which prevents sleep). In 1475, the world's first coffee shop was opened by Ottoman Turks in Constantinople.

New beliefs and customs always meet with resistance. Around 1530, when coffee first came to the attention of the Italians, a group of fanatical protestors complained in an audience with Pope Clement VII (formerly Giulio de' Medici) of the imminent dangers to all Christians of the "devil's beverage." The enlightened Florentine Pope first requested a sample of the offending brew. Upon taking a sip of the fragrant beverage, he decried that the true sin would be to permit only sinners access to the delicious liquid. He further declared that by his blessing, true believers could better defeat Satan by the use of coffee. Needless to say, that blessing fanned the flames of coffee consumption throughout Italy.

Dispersing widely into Europe via the port of Venice from around 1600, coffeehouses began to spring up in Italy. Captain John Smith, the founder of the Jamestown Colony in Virginia, first introduced coffee to the New World. By 1652, coffee had made its way to England. Coffeehouses came to be called "penny universities" because of the congregations of students and intellectuals who paid a penny to sip this congenial liquid. One of the early penny universities, Edward Lloyd's, attracted merchants and insurance brokers of England's sea trade amongst others, and eventually evolved into Lloyd's of London, the fabulously successful insurance company.

As an army of Turks marched to the doorstep of Vienna in 1675, Franz Georg Kolscheitzky managed to slip out of the city to bring relief forces, causing the Turks to flee. After their retreat, Kolschitzky claimed as his reward the sacks of coffee beans the Turks had left behind. He soon opened the first coffee house in Central Europe, further refining his coffee by filtering out the grounds, and sweetening it with milk. In 1690, a live coffee plant was smuggled out of the Arab port of Mocha by the Dutch, who transported it to Ceylon and their colony in the East Indies, Java. And 23 years later, the French smuggled a seedling to Martinique, where, by some 50 years afterwards, it had fathered 19 million coffee plants on this West Indian island. Nearly 80% of the world's coffee plants originated with this 1713 seedling.

A Brazilian coast guard officer, Francisco de Melo Palheta was dispatched by his country to arbitrate a border dispute in French Guiana in South America. He resolved the dispute between the French and Dutch, and in the meantime, struck up a torrid relationship with the wife of the governor of French Guiana. On his departure from his mission in 1727, Palheta was handed a bouquet by his paramour that contained coffee cuttings and seeds that were to initiate the Brazilian coffee industry.

Local roasting houses began a rapid decline in popularity in 1900 when Hills Bros. began packing roasted coffee in vacuum tins. By 1903, German researchers had developed a process of removing caffeine from coffee beans, while still maintaining the coffee flavor. This caffeine-less coffee was marketed under the brand name "Sanka." Two years later, Italians produced the first commercial espresso machine. The first drip coffeemaker was invented in 1908 by Melitta Bentz, who used blotting paper for the filter.

Thirty years later, the Nestlé Company came to the aid of the Brazilians to reduce their coffee glut with Nescafé instant coffee. By 1946, Achilles Gaggia had perfected his espresso machine. Its most famous product, Cappuccino, was named after the monks' robes of the Capuchin order, which shared its brownish color. Today coffee is second only to petroleum as the world's most-traded commodity, consumed at a rate of 400 billion cups a year, employing over 20 million people in its cultivation, production, shipping, packaging, and dispensing.

COFFEE THE DRUG

Nearly 90% of all Americans will consume caffeine in one form or another today. For over 50% of us, caffeine in the form of coffee, tea, cola, or chocolate will be ingested in quantities high enough (300 mg. per day) to suffer the secondary effects of these moderate drugs. Caffeine can produce nervousness, irritability, depression, insomnia, headaches, trembling, disorientation, and muscle tension. It is an addictive drug, operating in the same manner as heroin, cocaine, and amphetamines to stimulate the brain. If you feel that you need that next cup of coffee just like a heroin addict needs his next fix, you also are an addict.

When caffeine arrives in the brain, it immediately causes increased activity. Neurons fire off like a 4th of July display. The pituitary gland reacts by releasing hormones to stimulate the adrenal glands to pour out adrenaline (i.e., epinephrine). As a result, the pupils of your eyes dilate. Your blood pressure rises, due to the constriction of surface blood vessels, a decreased flow of blood to the stomach, and an increased heart rate. Your breathing tubes open up, and muscles tighten. The liver supplies extra emergency sugar to the bloodstream. All systems are on alert.

Caffeine stimulates increased dopamine levels in the brain, activating the pleasure centers just as heroin and cocaine do. Your brain soon comes to crave it, especially when the adrenaline begins to wear off, and fatigue and depression set in. The half life of caffeine is some 6 hours. That 200-milligram (mg.) dose you drink in your two late-afternoon cups of coffee is still at a disturbing level of 100 grams at midnight. When that sleep deficit slaps you in the face the next morning, you are likely to respond with more coffee, pulling your more deeply into the addictive cycle.

How high is your exposure to caffeine? If you drink a cup of brewed coffee, expect between 100 to 160 mg. of caffeine. Instant coffee yields between 50 to 75 mg. Decaffeinated coffee should contain no more that 4 mg. of caffeine per cup. Black tea contains between 20 to 50 mg. per cup, depending on the time you let it brew. Green tea is between 9 to 36 mg. Soft drinks like Coca-Cola, Dr. Pepper, Pepsi Cola, RC Cola, and Mountain Dew range from 33 to 65 mg. per 12-ounce serving. Surprisingly, baking chocolate contains up to 35 mg. per ounce. Even some non-prescription drugs contain significant quantities of caffeine. Excedrin has 65 mg. per tablet, and Anacin has over 30.

So, now that I am this caffeine addict, what am I to do? First, you must care. You must be concerned enough to discover, then put into motion, some realizable, concrete steps to your recovery. Be aware that coffee does not decrease the intoxicating effects of alcohol, nor does it relieve hangovers. That is a myth. Also, if you smoke, cut down or quit. Both habits increase your blood pressure, as well as causing acids to pour into your stomach.

Make a habit of keeping a diary where you note down your level of consumption, the conditions that make you consume more or less, your feelings, and the psychological and physical reactions you experience. Cut down your coffee intake to 2 cups a day. Substitute other non-caffeine drinks like hot cider, lemonade, or—best of all—a refreshing glass of water. Exercise. Walk, run, play tennis, ride a bike, or just make an excuse to get out. Eat regularly, focusing on healthy food. Educate those around you to reduce their caffeine intake. Where there is a will, there is a way.

THE NATURE OF TEA

Tea is obtained from the buds and leaves of an evergreen tree (*camellia sinensis*), which is usually trimmed to bush size. Once picked, the leaves must be dried quickly or they will "ferment" (actually a process of enzymatic oxidation), resulting in darkened leaves. Drying also prevents the formation of fungi.

White tea, highly prized in China, is produced by shielding new growth buds from sunlight, preventing the formation of chlorophyll. Green tea results when fresh growth is harvested, then dried by steam or in hot pans within one or two days of harvesting to prevent oxidation. Oolong tea, or blue-green tea, is allowed to oxidize from two to three days. Black tea (named for the color of the leaves), also known as red tea (named for the color of the prepared tea), is allowed to oxidize for two weeks up to a month. Black teas are named for the estate of origin, as well as their flush—first, second, or autumn. Their production is known as either orthodox, or CTC (i.e., crush, tear, curl). Some teas even undergo a second oxidation. A special winter tea popular in Japan as a health food is brewed from twigs and old leaves dry roasted over a fire.

As hot water is added to the tea, the leaves unfold ("the Agony of the Leaves"). The taste evolves as the myriad elements of the leaves enter into the water. Black tea should steep in boiling water (212° F.) for anywhere from thirty seconds up to five minutes before being strained and served. Green tea should be stewed in water of 175-185° F. For higher-quality leaves, the temperature can be even lower. Connoisseurs prefer adding the hot water to a pre-heated teapot. Oolong teas are best prepared with water heated to 195-212°F. The flavor is enhanced by using spring water. Premium teas are often steeped less than thirty seconds. Stirring is not recommended, nor squeezing the dregs from the teabag.

Some tea drinkers prefer adding milk to their tea to enhance the taste. Others enjoy adding lemon, sugar, honey or jam. In Tibet, yak butter and rock salt enhance their unique regional tea.

Tea bags were first used in 1908 when Thomas Sullivan began promoting his tea in small, reusable silk bags. Today these bags of "fannings" or "dust" are derided as an inferior byproduct of whole-leaf tea production. Tea bags have many drawbacks: the paper itself imparts an undesirable aftertaste;

when exposed to air, dried tea loses its flavored oils; and the bag prevents the tea from diffusing and steeping as it should. Employing a freeze-dry process, instant teas provide convenience at the cost of the delicate shades of flavor. Also, tea abhors refrigeration and freezing.

TEA'S EARLY HISTORY

Tea probably originated in northern Myanmar and the Chinese provinces of Yunnan and Sichnan. Legend has it that around 2737 BC, Shennong, the Chinese Emperor who purportedly invented agriculture and medicine, was boiling water to drink when a fortuitous wind blew some tea leaves into his bowl. It is historically recorded that by the first millennium BC, tea was being employed as a medicinal herb. Around 525 BC, Lao Tzu proclaimed this "froth of the liquid jade" as a quintessential element. Tea was not only renown for its medicinal properties, but also for its propensity for improving mental function. By 750 AD, tea was widespread in China. Tea bricks were commonly exchanged as currency.

In 1285, Marco Polo reported on the Chinese tea taxes. The first tea to arrive in Amsterdam came via China in the early seventeenth century. Tea became a fad in Paris in 1648. By 1689, camel caravans were making the year-long trek to Russia, loaded with the precious cargo. By the mid-seventeenth century, tea was being consumed in England's coffee houses, and from there soon reached the British Colonies. Today's greatest exporter of tea, India, greatly expanded its production under British rule. Adding milk and sugar to tea became customary there. The trail of tea eventually led from the India Tea Company to the Boston Tea Party.

TEA THE DRUG

Tea contains varying amounts of the amino acid theamine, the methylxanthines caffeine and theobromine, as well as polyphenolic antioxidant catechins. Theamine has proved effective in reducing mental and physical stress, as well as creating a sense of relaxation. Its use promotes the production of anti-bacterial proteins. Caffeine and theobromine are central nervous system stimulants—psychoactive substances—that promote heightened alertness. The greatest quantity of catechins are found in green and white tea. Expect to consume between thirty to ninety milligrams of caffeine per cup.

THE NATURE OF CHOCOLATE

Chocolate (or cocoa) is produced by fermenting, roasting, then grinding the beans of the tropical cacao tree, *Theobroma cacao*. The cacao beans from Central America were first widely traded by Olmec merchants from southern Mexico from the first millennium BC. The Mexica (popularly called Aztecs) named this drink *xocalatl*, "bitter water." The Mexica and Maya associated chocolate with their fertility goddesses. They flavored their royal drink with vanilla, ground chile, annatto, fruit and honey, and thickened it with a corn paste. Small bands of tribal-sponsored traders spread the beans throughout Mesoamerica, bartering up to one hundred cacao beans for a turkey, and as little as three beans for an avocado.

Currently, half of the world's cacao comes from Africa's Ivory Coast. These tropical trees grow only within twenty degrees of the equator, and with a minimum temperature of sixty degrees Fahrenheit. The most appreciated of the cacaos is the Criollo, which is found in the Caribbean, Central America and northern South America. Due to low yields and the difficulty in cultivating the tree, it is the scarcest and most expensive of the cacao beans. It is described by chocolate connoisseurs as possessing a "delicate yet complex" flavor with an enduring chocolate subtlety.

In the Amazon basin is found the Forastero, a hardier and higher yielding cacao tree, cultivated widely, as well as flourishing in the wild. It contains a strong chocolate essence, but of short duration, while lacking any subtle secondary flavors.

The third variety, the Trinitario, is a hybrid of the Criollo and the Forastero, originating in Trinidad.

CHOCOLATE PREPARATION

Once ripe, the cantaloupe-size pods are harvested, and the thirty or so beans with the pulp are fermented in piles or bins for three to seven days. They are then spread out in the sun and quickly dried to prevent the onset of mold. The beans then are roasted, graded and ground. The cocoa butter is removed, leaving the cocoa liquor. The cocoa liquor is then blended with cocoa butter, sugar and vanilla to create dark chocolate. By adding milk to this mixture, milk chocolate is created. Excluding the cocoa liquor results in white chocolate.

The final chocolate preparation should be stored at fifty-nine to sixty-three degrees Fahrenheit, with a humidity level below fifty percent. It is preferably stored in a dark place where it cannot absorb food odors.

CHOCOLATE THE DRUG

Chocolate consumption promotes the release of serotonin in the brain, which elicits a stream of pleasure. Brain activity and heart rate increase. The pleasure hormone, dopamine, floods the brain with the same trigger response as opiates. Dark chocolate is especially rich in the flavonoids epicatechin and gallic acid, which are believed to promote healthy hearts. Cocoa's antioxidants protect against LDL (low-density lipoprotein) oxidation. Eating chocolate mildly reduces blood pressure, but the downside is the inherent high fat content. Some seventy percent of the fat is stearic acid, a saturated fat, and oleic acid, an unsaturated fat. Yet serum LDL cholesterol levels are not raised by consuming chocolate. Also, it is believed that cocoa flavonoids are anticarcinogenic.

Chocolate contains the mood-affecting alkaloid, theobromine, a member of the same family as caffeine. Anandanide is an endogenous cannabinoid; tryptophan is a precursor to serotonin, which helps regulate moods; and phenethylamine is an endogenous amphetamine, which can trigger a release of endorphin in the brain. One ounce of bittersweet chocolate can contain from five to ten milligrams of caffeine. (A cup of coffee typically contains from one hundred to one hundred fifty milligrams of caffeine.)

Besides soothing and moistening the throat, chocolate contains the cough suppressant theobromine. Cocoa's flavonoids can inhibit diarrhea. Although chocolate is not a proven aphrodisiac, its phenethylamine can act as a sexual stimulant. Chocolate does not cause acne.

Unlike humans, animals cannot metabolize the theobromine in chocolate. It is toxic to dogs, cats, rodents, parrots, and even horses, potentially causing epileptic seizures, heart attacks, internal bleeding, and even death. Dark chocolate contains two to five times the concentration of theobromine as other chocolates. Carob serves as a desirable substitute for pet treats.

CONTENDING WITH COFFEE, TEA AND CHOCOLATE

Man is a chemical creature prone to excess. When doctors place a limit of 300 milligrams of caffeine intake per day, he exceeds that limit in search of the magic elixir that will convert his sleep-deprived brain to a hyperactive supercomputer. Energy drinks that enhance performance are pervasive. A friend, Mark, once noted that for every ounce of enhanced energy and euphoria a drug lends you, it insists on a 200% payback. After the euphoric high inevitably comes the crash. Overt hostility leads to confusion, disorientation, and even to paranoia, hallucinations, psychotic episodes, depression and seizures. Not a pretty sight. Like a steam locomotive madly rushing down the tracks, abuse of these drugs invites heart attacks and strokes.

Think. Stop to think. Consider pouring *half* a cup of coffee. Picture a glass of cool bubbling water, an effervescent fountain in an oasis, a joyful stream tumbling down an icy mountain crevasse. Try half a glass of water on the rocks. It is the quintessential liquid, the highest-octane stimulant known to mankind, but oh so subtle. Taste its essence, smell its sublime effervescence, feel its coolness, look into its other-dimensional transparency, listen to it flow out of your glass and into your physical being. Drink half a cup of tea, bite on a piece of melt-in-your-mouth chocolate, and then cleanse your mouth with pure water. Open your eyes, your senses—it really is divine.

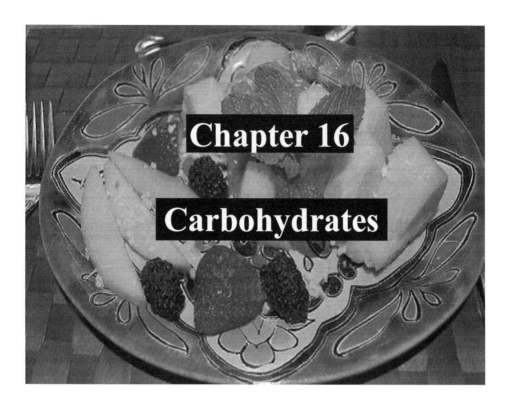

Chapter 16

Carbohydrates

WATER WITHIN

So just what is water? It exists all around us: in the air we breathe, the clouds that float above us, the rain that drenches the earth and flows in streams and rivers to the sea, the snow that caps mountains, eventually flowing in great glaciers into mountain valleys. And it is that same water that actually makes us fluid. It allows nutriments to follow an internal network of canals of veins, arteries and capillaries to every cell, also delivering the oxygen from our lungs so we can "burn" the food we eat to inherit the sun's energy trapped by photosynthesis. It returns the byproduct of this burning—carbon dioxide—back to the lungs to be exhaled. Our bloodstream is cleansed by the liver and kidneys to continue the infinite cycle of nutrition and cleansing, as well as bearing the cargo of messenger hormones and building-block hormones to constantly replace and repair body structures. All electrochemical processes rely on water's high electrical conductivity—a million times greater than any other naturally occurring liquid. 100 trillion cells intricately intertwined, interdependently laboring in harmony.

Muscle cells create movement large and small, nerve cells serve like an intricate phone network to allow near-instant communication from top to bottom, and organ cells control the delicate balance within each human—all faithfully, silently working, devoted to the good of the whole. With a world population of some 6 billion humans, *each* of us is composed of sufficient cells to distribute 16,000 cells to every other human on earth. The degree of interdependence, of cybernetic interconnectedness within each of us is staggering.

Each of us is a miniature ecosystem, an Internet of will, desire, hopes and dreams—in a floating sea of water. As you drink that glass of sparkling water before, after, and during, it becomes you, flows a million times through you, connecting every element of your body and spirit to the rivers and streams flowing through you. It allows you to recapture the surge of the intense energy of the sun to perform the thousands of complex tasks necessary to life—to move, to think, and ultimately, to dream.

PHOTOSYNTHESIS

The green chlorophyll in plants acts as a matchmaker, finding and aligning the perfect mates of carbon (C) and water (H_2O) that reside in the plant. Water can be easily absorbed from the ground or the air, and the CO_2 (the same CO_2 humans exhale as a waste product), is breathed in through tiny pores (stoma) on the leaves. As the sun's light bathes the plant, its energy becomes the prime mover, allowing an alignment and bonding of the carbon and the water to form a complex molecule of sugar. The sun's energy is literally trapped in the bound molecule—a family of atoms formed by 23 members (fructose—$C_5H_{12}O_6$), or 35 members (sucrose—$C_{12}H_{22}O_{11}$). When these bonds are eventually broken, as in digestion and assimilation, the freed energy of the sun converts into heat or kinetic energy at the disposal of the body to move muscles or race through neurons.

THE NATURE OF CARBOHYDRATES

Carbohydrates are a family of organic compounds that are essential in the maintenance of the life of plants and animals. Although plants alone have the capacity to assemble sugars, starches, and cellulose from carbon dioxide and water via photosynthesis, animals are totally dependent for their survival on these plant-manufactured compounds. Not only do they supply a continuous form of energy, but also perpetuate a form of stored chemical energy, as well as provide carbon atoms for the synthesis of cell components, even themselves becoming structural elements within the cells.

Carbohydrates (i.e., sugars, starches, and celluloses) were originally thought to be simply complexes of carbon (C) plus water (H_2O), yet other substances were discovered containing sulfur and nitrogen that had the same properties as the carbohydrates.

The most common of the simple sugars (i.e., monosaccharides) are glucose, fructose, galactose, and ribose. In solution, most glucose molecules ($C_6H_{12}O_6$) appear in the form of a ring:

Sugars like D-glucose ($C_6H_{12}O_6$) and sucrose ($C_{12}H_{22}O_{11}$) are readily soluble, sweet, and crystalline. Starches ($C_6H_{10}O_5$)n are colloidal and accumulate into paste. They are either amylose—long, unbranched chains of glucose, or amylopectin—a highly branched network of 24-to-30 glucose molecules. Cellulose ($C_6H_{10}O_5$)n is insoluble. It is composed of long, unbranched chains of glucose molecules.

Sucrose is an oligosaccharide, found in cane sugar, beet sugar, maple sap, and honey, as well as a wide variety of fruits, seeds, flowers, and roots. Its formula ($C_{12}H_{22}O_{11}$) can be visualized as:

t

creation of energy-rich bonds, principally the pyrophosphate bond of the coenzyme adenosinetriphosphate (ATP).

The simple sugars, monosaccharides, cannot be hydrolyzed into simpler substances. Oligosaccharides—compound sugars—are products of condensation of two-to-five molecules of simple sugars that can be hydrolyzed. Polysaccharides—glycogen, starch, and cellulose—are tasteless, nonreducing, amorphous agglomerations that yield a high number of monosaccharide molecules by hydrolysis. Because humans and other members of the mammalian family do not possess cellulose-decomposing microorganisms in their intestinal tracts capable of digesting cellulose, it passes through the intestinal tract as unprocessed fiber.

Certain disaccharides and polysaccharides resist absorption into the intestine. They are digested (i.e., hydrolyzed) first by enzymes, glycosidases, and then pass through the intestinal mucosa, to be subsequently escorted through the surrounding tissue, and then into the bloodstream. These sugars are then absorbed by the liver and stored as glycogen. As necessary, the liver releases glucose into the bloodstream.

CALORIES

A calorie is a unit of heat energy. If you take a slice of bread, dry it out, place a container with 1 gram of H_2O above it, then set the bread on fire, the flames will heat up the water. For every degree Centigrade of rise in temperature, the bread has released 1 calorie of heat energy. If you heat 100 grams of water 30° C., the caloric input is 3,000 calories (100 times 30), or 3 Calories (1,000 calories, with a small "c" = 1 kilocalorie = 1 Calorie, with a capital "C").

Before you dip into that bag of cookies, consider the amount of calories per ounce: 138 calories (kilocalories are commonly referred to simply as "calories" with a small "c"). That cinnamon bun smiling at you from your plate, will melt in your mouth, soon depositing 110 calories into your blood-stream. That friendly little muffin will deliver 86 calories to your body. An ounce of soft pretzels weighs in at 82 calories, and that innocent slice of white bread, 73.

Compare your caloric intake above with a plump little potato at 26 calories. A phosphorous-rich banana contains 25 calories. An ounce of oatmeal only delivers 19, while promising to lower your bad cholesterol, LDL (low density lipoprotein). An apple (14 calories per ounce) and carrots (11 calories per ounce) are healthy alternatives, as is broccoli (9 calories per ounce). Romaine lettuce, with no additives, is an attractive 5 calories per ounce. Pick and choose. Stop. Think. Then pick and choose wisely. Your health, happiness—your life depend on the choices you make.

Celebrate with an aperitif: a tall crystal glass of clear, wondrous water. Take a bite of healthy food, chew to enjoy, swallow, and then rinse your mouth with a cascade of pure water. Feel the cleanliness, the freshness of an after-dinner drink of H_2O. Heartburn, headache, and fatigue all gradually fade as you follow a common-sense approach. You are what you eat. You are what you drink. You make conscious choices. And as your choices become healthy habits, your body strengthens, and your mind clears. Take a step at a time.

Congratulations. You have chosen the path to success.

INSULIN

The pancreas, discovered by Herophilus (335-280 BC), a Greek anatomist and surgeon, is an abdominal organ located just below the stomach. It plays a double role: (1) exocrine (i.e., a gland secreting externally), producing digestive enzymes, as well as (2) endocrine (i.e., a gland producing hormones), secreting hormones like insulin, glucagon, and somatosatin.

Once secreted into the bloodstream, insulin circulates until it finds a home in an individual cell. This implanted insulin then facilitates the absorption of passing glucose. When, for some reason, the pancreas malfunctions and cannot release sufficient insulin to act as the gatekeeper for the cells, the excess sugars meandering through the bloodstream begin to wreak havoc. This is the case of diabetes.

The imbalance of hormones spewed out by the placenta of pregnant women can result in a shortage of insulin. To minimize the potential danger, a low-carbohydrate diet is recommended, accompanied by careful blood-sugar monitoring. This monitoring is generally accomplished by pricking the finger to extract a drop of blood. Once in contact with a monitor, the drop of blood prompts a numerical readout to appear, representing glucose saturation. This is normally done fasting before breakfast, then two hours after beginning each meal.

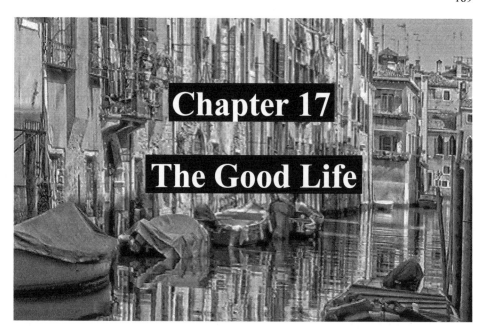

Chapter 17

The Good Life

OVERVIEW

Anticipate your future state of being. If you sense you soon will be in need of hydration, drink a tall glass of water before your thirst screams at you. Keep a bottle of water at hand, at home, in the office, and in your car. Take a sip—then listen to your body to see if you might want another sip. Finish up activities with a glass of water. Keep yourself fresh. Maintain balance in your life. Provide yourself with healthy options: an interesting, appealing variety of fruits, a rainbow display of vegetables, and lean meats. Be creative while shopping, choosing a wide variety of foods. Appreciate the food you prepare, savor it as you eat, and serve yourself judiciously. Then seek out moderate physical activity to keep your body in rhythm. Discover your own personal equilibrium —somewhere between eating to live and living to eat.

Create a balanced diet. Focus on a pleasant variety of fruits and vegetables. Include a portion of protein-rich foods. Decorate your table with a fruit basket, while steering clear of

190

refined carbohydrates like baked goods, white breads, and pastas.

When buying and preparing protein foods, choose amongst beans, nuts, soy products, fish, and skinless chicken.

Sprinkle less salt on your food. Taste each preparation first without salt, and then add a minimum amount to your satisfaction. Check labels for sodium content.

If you drink alcoholic beverages, do so in moderation. More is not better. If one drink relaxes you, do not automatically assume ten additional drinks will lend you ten times the pleasure. They will not. If such were the case, we would spend our days on Ferris wheels and roller coasters, consuming sodas and ice cream cones until we burst with pleasure. Food and drink are a continuum of ups and downs—a wave that brings most pleasure when ridden with proper proportion and common sense.

Explore the variety of water that awaits your discovery: on the rocks, room temperature, bubbling with natural gas, permeated with CO_2, pre-meal, appetizer, post-meal, energizer, pre-exercise, mid-exercise, post-exercise, midnight thirst quencher, morning awakener, healthy chaser, substitute supreme, toast to all occasions, etc.

MEAL SUGGESTIONS

Try cutting up fresh fruit and presenting a mixed bowl on the table where it will call attention to itself. Fresh fruits like apples, pears, and bananas will not turn brown if you mix them with acidic fruits like oranges, grapefruit, or pineapples. Favor the selection of fruits high in potassium like watermelon, bananas, cantaloupe, peaches, oranges, apricots, and prunes. Also, dried fruits can be easily stored and are always on hand. A vegetable tray of cut-up raw cauliflower, broccoli, celery, and green and red peppers make an appealing, uplifting decoration. Serve them with dip or salad dressing.

A good selection of frozen vegetables can be easily stored and prepared in a jiffy in your microwave oven. Ditto with frozen fruit—in an instant it can be in a bowl to enliven a meal or a mid-meal snack. Offer frozen fruit bars (the pure-fruit variety) as a special dessert, or try pudding prepared with low-fat milk. When about to prepare wheat-based cookies, pancakes, waffles, or muffins, set aside the wheat flour and instead use rice flour. You will be amazed and delighted at this light, healthy substitute.

Prepare that after-meal coffee latte or cappuccino with low-fat milk. It will be just as delicious, but markedly better for you.

Make your heart happy by feasting on fatty fish at least once a week. Grill it or broil it. Try a salad with olive oil and vinegar. Read, research, and use your imagination to discover the world of soy products. Chew on some nuts. Drink a glass of grape juice to reduce the risk of blood clots. Sip on a delicious cup of black tea. And don't allow yourself to forget your ever-present fountain of youth and vitality—H_2O.

Tomatoes reduce the risk of prostate cancer. Green tea also inhibits cancer. Many other foods have highly beneficial effects. Yogurt aids the digestive tract, while cranberry juice helps prevent urinary-tract infections. Oats lower LDL and total cholesterol levels. Dairy products and other calcium-fortified foods reduce the risk of osteoporosis. Healthy vision is maintained by the consumption of carrots, collard greens, kale, and spinach. You merely have to reach out to live sensibly—buy a wide variety of foods, prepare and serve them with gusto, then enjoy.

Here's to your health and happiness!

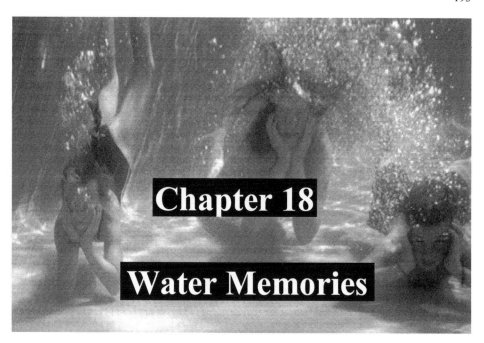

Chapter 18

Water Memories

JUNGLE

We lay quiet, staring up at the black abyss of the heavens from deep within a steaming tropical hut, a steady downpour dancing off the thatch roof, draining in rivulets past the screened windows. A magic music enveloped us as the ebony sky drained ceaselessly through the night. Palms shrugged their wet shoulders beneath the fluid weight of the rain, spilling the liquid sky onto huge umbrella leaves below, then onto the jungle floor, scurrying into the thousand streamlets to steamy waterways that hurried out to the sea.

RIVER

Animated children ran at the river from its grassy banks, yelping and leaping high to splash heavily into the chocolate flow. Rising to the surface, blowing out bursts of joy, striking at the reflective surface, leaving tiny whirlpools in their wake as they struggled onto the shore, water leaping and hurtling onto the wet sand. They shook their hair and a shower of glistening beads fell about them like a halo.

THUNDERSTORM

A foreboding wall of clouds as tall as the heavens swept broadly across the plains, roiling and billowing as the storm front attacked. Gusts of wet wind bent the trees sideways, impressing us with nature's might. Lightning leapt out of the massive cloudbank in a streak of light that illuminated the monster. Heavy thunder rumbled past us. Then the deluge hit. A leaden curtain of water enveloped us, splashing vigorously off the ground. We ran for shelter, and then stared at the drenched landscape as wave after wave of the dense rain cascaded down.

Suddenly, nickel-size hail began to pelt the lawn, leaping up vigorously as if emerging from the grass to escape the earth. The sky turned an ethereal emerald green, and the wind subsided, then it was virtually still. We raced out to gather up a few beads of ice and tossed them into our mouths, laughing uproariously. The ice pellets felt warm as they melted into oblivion and were swallowed, filling us with the seeds of the storm.

IGLOO

Fat, lazy snowflakes whirled down from a faded blue sky onto our sleeves. We scooped up a fistful of snow and took a careful bite like cotton candy. It melted deliciously, freezing our tongues. On hands and knees, we crawled into our igloo, sculptured from a hardened snowdrift in our back yard. We lay on our backs on the packed snow, listening to the insistent whining wind whirling about our ice fortress. The huge cakes of frozen snow above us were bordered in a heavenly luminescent blue. Our breath flowed out in slow white puffs. We pulled icicles from the freezer we had carved into the snow wall. They were like wondrous white Popsicles that nourished our thirst. We, ourselves, had melted into the winter in our timeless white bubble, drinking in the frozen eternal moment.

SWIMMING POOL

We rode our bikes to the park, changed into our swimming suits, and ran diving into the inviting coolness of the pool. Staccato voices bounced off the choppy surface, facets of sky, faces and trees reflecting summer's joy. Holding our breath, we dove deep into the liquid blue as effortlessly as dolphins, and chased the waves as we madly fled from the desperate dunkings and the slapping tags. Our hands scooped up brash curtains of water as we wildly splashed one another.

We were frolicking fish in a mad escapade, darting about a weightless, buoyant world. As we jumped up out of the pool to seek out our sun-tanning schoolmates, our skin began to shiver as the glistening coating of water evaporated and cooled us. We gulped down a few mouthfuls of refreshing water from the drinking fountain, and then went off chasing the breeze. Bright, billowing clouds played out scenes from cartoons and mythology, as butterflies fluttered and bees buzzed about.

GARDEN

The long, green hose bent like a sleeping snake across the lawn. A frivolous stream of water came gushing out, until my thumb clamped down and converted it into a rainbow spray. The flowers perked up at the sudden cloudburst of cool rainbow water, and smiled happily at me.

A soft song escaped my lips. Water is life. Water is energy. It is the magic elixir that sends currents of love flowing down through the earth, up through my garden, and on up to the billowing clouds, then gently down again in torrents of nourishing rain. I unclamped my thumb and lifted the hose to let the water easily arc into the air. I bent over to let it course through my open lips, drinking deeply of its life-giving force. I began awakening like my garden, smiling at the delight of it all. I felt blessed.

MINERAL SPRINGS

We had crossed lush pine mountains to descend onto the barren desert valley. Soon our bodies were effortlessly submerging into the warm mineral springs of therapeutic waters. Suspended effortlessly in the buoyant liquid, I rinsed my mouth out with the sweet water, feeling its robust flow within and without. Looking out across the baking desert through the chimerical heat waves, I gazed at the pageant of stoic brown-and-green survivors still and patient, awaiting a promised summer shower to explode for a brief moment into a curtain of yellow, purple and red blossoms.

The swirling bath suspended us in a timeless dimension where worries, preoccupations and responsibilities melted away like mirages. We were one with the insistent flow of nature. I drank deeply of the fragrant mineral waters, and stared into the azure sky where wisps of clouds lazily floated by.

MOUNTAIN RETREAT

We had driven up the winding mountain road through sentinel pines, through the pungent perfume of the forest, to a retreat where the world sat still. We reclined within a rustic cabin restaurant at a weathered table, pouring marvelously effervescent spring water into our glasses. We toasted the moment. Through the open door of the restaurant, up over the stone path, crept the fog. It was a fairy tale. The mist gently twisted like a phantom lizard, cautiously entering the open door, hugging the cool tile floor, and then evaporating into the Netherlands as it approached the crackling blaze in the fireplace. We looked at one another, amazed. We laughed. As we lifted our glasses, the joyful water bubbled, and then tickled our throats. I paused to ponder on the significant simplicity of nature.

TEARS

My sister had been accepted by a college far, far away. She who nourished me and cherished me must sever our magic bond. Tears welled up at the finality and profundity of my loss. They overflowed, draining down over my cheeks and onto my lips. As they touched my tongue, a warm, salty sensation flowed through me. I was a sea of salty water, primeval and sublime. I had touched my soul.

It had been an eternity in limbo, but my sister was at last home for Christmas vacation. The world was ablaze with festive food, bright lights, white snow-sledding days, and candle-lit nights of tales and laughter. My eyes overflowed with joy, and as I again tasted my salty tears and once again touched my soul's essence, I realized that pain and joy flow from the same fountain. I lifted my crystal glass to my lips and rejoiced at the vital fluid that coursed through me.

ICE SKATING

The lake had frozen solid. I lay spread-eagled across its smooth surface, staring down at the white air bubbles trapped far below within the black ice. My bare hands caressed its glassy surface, and I sensed its smoothness and warmth. Back on my feet again, I effortlessly skated off into infinity. The shore seemed somehow days away. A cool breeze flirted with my hair, and bathed my face. I was lost between the cobalt sky and the deep, deep ebony waters just beneath my skates. I glided through the air. "This must be heaven on earth," I thought.

BLIZZARD

I had come out to trudge through the blizzard, to thrust myself into the heart of nature's fury. The driving white ice stung my eyes and froze my cheeks. Dim streetlamps were glowing eerily yellow like lost moons. Bent forward against the elements, I plowed ahead, the drifting snow swirling in and around my footprints, erasing my steps as soon as I lifted my feet to leave them behind. I bent into the future. As I opened my mouth to gulp in the frozen air, a swirl of snowflakes invaded my being. Swallowing the storm, I staggered into its fury a few steps more, then turned with the insistent wind at my back filling my sails, and set course for home. The wind swirled and wailed at me to quickly make my way. Yet I was at that moment already at home, forever trudging through the dimensionless, relentless blizzard.

CLIFF DIVING

We bounced over the frisky waves in our aluminum outboard skiff, racing toward the horizon where the cliffs soared far above the lake. Once ashore, we ascended the narrow trail through lush foliage to the harrowing drop down to the amber water far below. It was deep, inviting, and frightening. The leap of faith, a haunting current of air violently rushing by, then the iron surface of the water. Crash! Our bodies broke the mirror surface, exploding up jets of vaporized water slamming into our faces. My legs stung. I was suddenly in a watery tomb, deep within the lake. Silence. Then a flurry of bubbles urged me to the surface, slowly lifting me up towards the sun. I began to stroke at the water, wildly, desperately upward. My lungs exploded, and then gasped in a deep breath of air.

BODY SURFING

A long, deep-throated roar preceded the waves that attacked the beach from far out in the ocean. Five-foot walls of water rose, then scurried toward the shore, madly stirring up white foam and sand before crashing at our feet. We strode out into the raging surf, and then dived into the oncoming wave. Its turbulent force rotated furiously just beneath us, then left us stranded in shallow waters. We moved forward, repeatedly diving deeper into the sea. At last we were floating free, surging up, bobbing in the tumultuous breakers. A series of three extraordinary waves loomed on the horizon, blocking out half the sky.

As we turned and swam towards shore, the first wave overcame us. We flattened our bodies, paddled furiously, and then bent over the churning dynamo. It lifted us up before it and shot us forward, our bodies suspended, perpetually sliding down the face of the advancing wave. It soon spent itself, leaving us gasping for breath far from where we had mounted its fury. Our skin glistened, our hair permeated with fine sand. The next wave slapped at our legs, then ran on ahead to slide peacefully up onto the beach. Ebb and tide.

We raced up to our towels, and each of us pulled out a sweating bottle of water from our ice chest. As the remnants of the surf drained off our bodies, we tipped our heads back and drank deeply of the invigorating water. It satiated our thirst and refreshed our senses. And then we turned to battle the incessant waves once again.

It's all about water.

"A journey of a thousand miles must begin with a single step."

—Lao-tzu

BIBLIOGRAPHY

"Ask the Expert." 2 Sept. 2001 <http://www.my
      primetime.com> (2 Sept. 2001).

Aswartz, and Beadmomsw. "The History of Alcohol."
      <http://www.get.theinfo.org/alcohol1> (10 Sept. 2001).

Bartlett, John. *Familiar Quotations.* Ed. Emily Morison Beck.
      Boston: Little, Brown and Company, 1982.

Borio, Gene. "Tobacco Timeline." <http://www.tobacco.org>
      (3 Sept. 2001).

Bowra, C.M. *Classical Greece.* New York: Time
      Incorporated, 1965.

"Brain Nutritional Deficits." <http://www.open.org/~tahana/
      ADA/twfbrdef.htm> (2 Aug. 2001).

"Breaking the Code of Food Labels." <http://www.heartinfo.
      org> (2 Sept. 2001).

"The Brewing Industry and Prohibition." <http:www.history.
      ohio-state.edu/projects/prohibition/brewing/> (16 Sept.
      2001).

"Caffeine." 20 July 1998. <http://www.mckinley.uiuc.
      edu/health-info/drug-alc/caffeine.heml> (27 Sept. 2001).

"Can physical activity reduce my chances of getting a heart
      attack?" 22 Jan. 2001 <http:www.nih.gov> (3 Sept.
      2001).

Casson, Lionel. *Ancient Egypt.* New York: Time
      Incorporated, 1965.

"Chemistry of Caffeine." <http://www.geocities.com/
      CapeCanaveral/Launchpad/6202/che.htm> (27 Sept.
      2001).

"Chocolate." 9 May 2007 <http://en.widkpedia.org/wiki/
      Chocolate> (14 May 2007).

"Cigarettes and Other Nicotine Products." <http://www.drug
      abuse.gov> (3 Sept. 2001).

"Coffee History." 30 Mar. 2000. <http://www.koffeekorner.

204

com/koffeehistory.htm> (27 Sept. 2001).

"Coffee History, Cultivation, Botanical Notes." <http:// sovrana.com/libstory.htm> (Sept. 2001).

Concise Encyclopedia of Science & Technology. 3rd ed. New York: McGraw-Hill, Inc., 1992.

Condor, Bob. "Weight Up." *Wisconsin State Journal.* August 22, 2001, sec. B:1-2.

"Diet Tips." <http://www.1800DietFoods.com> (2 Sept. 2001).

"Do we get enough exercise from our daily activities?" <http: www.nih.gov> (3 Sept. 2001).

"Don't Stop the Fiber Intake." <http://www.medformation. com> (18 Aug. 2001).

"Effective ways to avoid injuries." <http://www.nih.gov> (3 Sept. 2001).

"An Egg a Day." <http://www.medformation.com> (18 Aug. 2001).

Erowid. "Alcohol Timeline." 2001 <http://www.erowid.org/ chemicals/alcohol/alcohol_timeline.php3> (10 Sept. 2001).

"Everybody Needs a Little Fat." <http://www.medformation. com> (18 Sept. 2001).

"Exercise." <http://www.americanheart.org> (2 Sept. 2001).

"Exercise Essentials." <http:www.acefitness.org> (22 Aug. 2001).

"Fad Diets: The Kernel of Truth." <http://www.medformation. com> (18 Aug. 2001).

Family Medical Guide. Ed. Charles B. Clayman, MD. New York: Random House, 1994.

"Fatty Acids." <http://www.medformation.com> (18 Aug. 2001).

"Fetal alcohol effect (FAE) and syndrome (FAS)." 2001. <http:www. findarticles.com/cf_dis/g2699/0004/ 2699000467/pl/article.jhtml> (10 Sept. 2001).

"Fetal alcohol syndrome." 1999. <http://www.findarticles.

com/cf_dis/g2601?0005?2601000536/pl/article.jhtml>
(10 Sept. 2001).

"Fiber Can Lower Cholesterol." <http://www.medformation.
com> (18 Sept. 2001).

"Fish to Reduce Stroke Risk." <http://www.medformation.
com> (18 Aug. 2001).

"Food Diary for IBS." <http://www.medformation.com>
(18 Aug. 2001).

"Foods to Prevent Cancer." <http://www.medformation.com>
(18 Aug. 2001).

Grieger, Lynn, RD, CD, CDE. "Greens." <http://www.heart
info.org> (2 Sept. 2001).

---. "Phytochemicals and Legumes." <http://www.heartinfo.
org> (2 Sept. 2001).

Hadas, Moses. *Imperial Rome.* New York: Time
Incorporated, 1965.

Hark, Lisa, Ph.D., R.D. "Defining Saturated, Poly, Mono and
Trans Unsaturated Fats." <http://www.heartinfo.org>
(31 Aug. 2001).

---. "Distinguishing Between Hunger and Food Cravings."
<http://www.heartinfo.org> (31 Aug. 2001).

---. "A Grocery List and Meal Plan Helps With Weight Loss."
<http://www.heartinfo.org> (31 Aug. 2001).

---. "USDA Survey Tracks Americans' Eating Habits."
<http://www.heartinfo.org> (31 Aug. 2001).

Hayes, Jack. "Dr. John S. Pemberton (Inventor of Coca-Cola)."
<http://memory.loc.gov/ammem/ccmphtml/colainvnt.
html> (28 July 2001).

"Healthy Meat Eating." <http://www.medformation.com>
(18 Aug. 2001).

Hernan, Alice, MS, RD. "MyPyramid Steps to a Healthier
You." <http://mypyramid.gov> (28 May 2007).

"The History of Coffee." <http://www.telusplanet.net/
public/coffee/history.htm> (27 Sept. 2001).

"How Caffeine Works." <http://www.howstuffworks.

206

com/caffeine.htm> (27 Sept. 2001).

"How do different activities help my heart and lungs?"
<http:www.nih.gov> (3 Sept. 2001).

"How do I keep going?" <http:www.nih.gov> (3 Sept. 2001).

Huskey, Robert J. "Babies and the 'Blues.'" 27 July 2001
<http://www.people.Virginia.edu/~rjh9u/crhblues.html>.

"Jamaican Coffee—the finest in the world!" 1 June 2001.
<http:www.chem..uwimona.edu.jm:1104/lectures/
coffee.html> (27 Sept. 2001).

"The Joy of Soy." <http://www.medformation.com> (18 Aug.
2001)

Kight, Juli. <http://herbsforhealth.about.com/library/weekly/
aal112197.htm?once=true&> (24 July 2001).

Lemonick, Michael D. and Alice Park. "The Science of
Addiction." *Time.* July 16, 2007: 42-48.

"Making Nutrition a Habit." <http://www.medformation.com>
(18 Aug. 2001).

Modern Nutrition in Health and Disease. 8th ed. Eds. Maurice
E. Shils, M.D., Sc.D., James A. Olson, Ph.D., and Moshe
Shike, M.D. Philadelphia: Lea & Febiger, 1994.

Moore, Sylvia A., PhD, RD, FADA, and Janice G. Smith, BS.
OBGYN.net. <http://www.obgyn.net/femalepatient/
default/asp?page=moore_tfp> (27 July 2001).

"My Food Plan." Minneapolis: International Diabetes Center,
2004.

"Nuts Can Be Good for You." <http://www.medformation.
com> (18 Aug. 2001).

"Orange and Tangerine Juices." <http://www.medformation.
com> (18 Aug. 2001).

The Oxford Companion to Classical Civilization. Ed. Simon
Hornblower, and Antony Spawforth. New York: The
Oxford University Press, 1998.

"Pancreas." 5 May 2007. <http://en.wikipedia.org/wiki/
Pancreas> (23 May 2007).

Parker, Sybil P., ed., et al. "Fructose." *Concise Encyclopedia of*

Science & Technology. 3rd ed. New York: McGraw-Hill, Inc., 1992.

---. "Sucrose." *Concise Encyclopedia of Science & Technology.* 3rd ed. New York: McGraw-Hill, Inc., 1992.

"Prohibition." *The New Encyclopaedia Britannica, vol. 9.* Chicago: Encyclopaedia Britannica, Inc., 1986.

"Prohibition in the 1920s." 6 May 1998. <http://www.geo cities.com/Athens/Troy/4399/> (16 Sept. 2001).

"Research Wrap-up: Exercise and Distress." <http:www. acefitness.org> (22 Aug. 2001).

Ronzio, Robert A. *The Encyclopedia of Nutrition & Good Health.* New York: Facts on File, Inc., 1997.

"Senior Fitness." <http://www.vidbook.com> (2 Sept. 2001).

Sherwood, Lauralee. *Human Physiology.* 2nd. ed. New York: West Publishing Company, 1993.

Shils, Maurice E., James A. Olson, and Moshe Shike, eds. *Modern Nutrition in health and disease.* 8th ed. 2 vols. Malvern, PA: Lea & Febiger, 1994.

Shute, Nancy. "Over the Limit?" U.S. News & World Report 23 April 2007: 60-68.

"Take Steps to Prevent Diabetes." <http://www.medformation. com> (18 Aug. 2001).

"Tea." 14 May 2007. <http://en.wikipedia.org/wiki/Tea> (14 May 2007).

Two sample activity programs. <http:www.nih.gov> (3 Sept. 2001).

Vallee, Bert L., M.D. "Alcohol in the Western World: A History." <http:www.beckmanwine.com/prevtopx.htm> (10 Sept. 2001).

Velasco, M., and N. Caporaso. "Dopamine: Pharmacologic and Therapeutic Aspects." 1 Jan. 1998 <http://www. biopsychiatry.com/dopapharm.htm> (9 Sept. 2001).

Webster's New World Dictionary. Ed. Victoria Neufeldt, and

208

David B. Guralnik. New York: Simon & Schuster, Inc.,
    1991.
"A well-balanced diet." <http://dietadvice.homestead.com>
    (18 Aug. 2001).
"What is a Serving." <http://www.medformation.com>
    (18 Aug. 2001).
"What is a Well-Balanced Diet?" <http://www.medformation.
    com> (18 Aug. 2001).
Whitehouse, Ruth, and John Wilkins. The Making of
    Civilization. New York: Alfred A. Knopf, 1986.
"Why Prohibition?" <http:www.cohums.ohio-state.edu/
    /history/projects/prohibition/whyprohibition.htm> (16
    Sept. 2001).
"Wine." 2000. <http://www.encarta.msn.com/find/print.asp?
    &pg=8&ti=0634D000&sc=13&pt=1> (10 Sept. 2001).

Made in the USA
Lexington, KY
07 February 2015